Cardiology pocket

M000191704

Author:

Debabrata Mukherjee, MD, FACC
Chief, Cardiovascular Medicine
Professor of Internal Medicine
Vice Chairman
Department of Internal Medicine
Texas Tech University
4800 Alberta Avenue El Paso, Tx 79905

Acknowledgments:

Anthony Bavry, MD, MPH
Director, Gainesville VA Medical Center
Catheterization Laboratory Assistant
Professor of Medicine
Division of Cardiovascular Medicine
University of Florida Gainesville, FL 32610

Acknowledgments:

Raghuraman Vidhun, MD, FACC
Cardiology Associates of Waterbury
455 Chase Parkway
Waterbury, CT 06708

Andreas Ruß, MD
Internal Medicine Specialist
Kirchplatz 1
83734 Hausham, Germany

Editing: Carla Knobloch, MD, Andrea Raunecker, MD
Cover Illustration: Alexander Storck, Ekaterina Zenz
Production: Alexander Storck, Petra Rau
Publisher: Börm Bruckmeier Publishing LLC, www.media4u.com

Printed in China through Colorcraft Ltd., Hong Kong
ISBN 978-1-59103-252-6

Preface

Cardiology is a dynamic field with rapid changes in management strategy and technology. The advent of newer technology presents both an opportunity as well as numerous challenges for the practitioner to treat patients optimally.

The succinct **Cardiology Pocketbook** aims to provide clinicians with concise, easily accessible guidance on important and commonly seen cardiology conditions. The pocket book features evidence-based discussion on optimal use of commonly performed diagnostic tests in the field of cardiology. It includes information about cardiac symptomatology, ischemic heart disease, cardiomyopathies, arrhythmias, heart failure, and vasculitides.

The pocket book should help guide cardiologists in selecting the optimal diagnostic tool for each cardiologic condition. This pocket book also provides guidance of preoperative evaluation of patients, taking into account specific risk factors and comorbidities, and reviews commonly used drugs by cardiologists. Highly practical in format, content, and style, **Cardiology Pocketbook** should serve as a succinct, yet comprehensive, easily accessible point-of-care reference for busy practitioners and cardiology trainees. Tools such as treatment algorithms, tables, and illustrations make this volume a practical reference tool.

Debabrata Mukherjee, MD, FACC
Chief, Cardiovascular Medicine
Texas Tech University Health Sciences Center

4 Contents

1 Symptoms and Presentation

1.1 Chest Pain

1.1.1 Cardiovascular

Possible Diagnosis	Symptoms/Characteristics	Diagnostic Procedures
Myocardial ischemia (acute MI/ unstable angina/ stable angina)	• Chest discomfort with or without radiation to the arm(s), back, neck, jaw, or epigastrum • Shortness of breath, weakness, diaphoresis, nausea, lightheadedness • S_4 gallop • Sometimes late systolic murmur	• Serial ECGs and cardiac markers • Stress imaging test considered in patients with non-diagnostic ECG findings and no cardiac marker elevation • Often heart catheterization and coronary angiography if findings are suggestive of coronary disease
Thoracic aortic dissection	• Sudden tearing pain radiating to the back • Syncope, stroke, leg ischemia • Asymmetric blood pressure or pulses • Tachycardia, bradycardia, hypotension • Diaphoresis, confusion, ashen color	• Chest Radiography • CT angiography of aorta • Transthoracic or transesophageal echocardiography
Pericarditis	• Sharp pain (constant or intermittent) • Pain aggravated by breathing or swallowing food • Pain relief by sitting leaning forward	• ECG • Cardiac markers • Echocardiography • MRI/MRA
Myocarditis	• Fever, dyspnea, fatigue, chest pain • Recent infection (viral or other) • Sometimes findings of heart failure	• ECG and cardiac markers • ESR • C-reactive protein • Echocardiography

1.1.2   Gastrointestinal

Possible Diagnosis	Symptoms/Characteristics	Diagnostic Procedures
Esophageal rupture	• Sudden severe pain following vomiting or instrumentation (e.g. esophagogastroscopy) • Subcutaneous crepitus • Asymmetric breath sounds • Tachycardia, bradycardia, hypotension • Diaphoresis, confusion, ashen color	• Chest Radiography • Esophagography • CT scan
Pancreatitis	• Epigastric or lower chest pain (worsened when lying flat, relieved by leaning forward) • Vomiting and abdominal tenderness • Shock • History of alcohol abuse or biliary tract disease	• Serum amylase and lipase • Abdominal CT
Peptic ulcer	• Recurrent, vague epigastric or right upper quadrant discomfort in a patient who smokes or uses alcohol excessively • Relieved by food, antacids, or both	• Clinical evaluation • Endoscopy • Sometimes testing for *Helicobacter pylori*
Esophageal reflux (GERD)	• Recurrent burning pain radiating from epigastrium to throat • Exacerbated by bending down or lying down • Relieved by antacids	• Clinical evaluation • Endoscopy • Motility studies
Biliary tract disease	• Recurrent or right upper quadrant discomfort to following meals	• Ultrasonography of the gallbladder
Esophageal motility disorders	• Pain (insidious onset, long-standing, may accompany swallowing)	• Barium swallow

1.1.3 Pulmonary

Possible Diagnosis	Symptoms/Characteristics	Diagnostic Procedures
Pulmonary embolism	• Pleuritic pain • Dyspnea, tachycardia, sometimes fever • Hemoptysis, shock	• CT angiography • VQ scan • Doppler or duplex study of extremities showing positive findings of Deep Vein Thrombosis
Tension pneumothorax	• Significant dyspnea, hypotension, unilateral diminished breath sounds and hyperresonance to percussion • Sometimes subcutaneous air	• Usually clinical • Chest Radiography
Pneumonia	• Fever, chills, cough, purulent sputum • Dyspnea, tachycardia	• Chest Radiography
Pneumothorax	• Sometimtes unilateral diminished breath sounds • Subcutaneous air • May follow injury or occur spontaneously (especially in tall, thin patients or patients with COPD)	• Chest Radiography
Pleuritis	• Pain with breathing, cough • May have preceding pneumonia, pulmonary embolism, or viral infection	• Clinical evaluation

1.1.4 Other

Musculoskeletal chest wall pain	• Pain typically persistent • Worsened with passive or active motion • Diffuse or focal tenderness	• Clinical evaluation
Various thoracic cancers	• Sometimes chronic cough • Weight loss and fever	• Chest Radiography • Chest CT • Bone-scintigraphy
Herpes zoster	• Linear vesicular rash • Band-like pain unilaterally midthorax	• Clinical evaluation
Idiopathic	• Various features	• Diagnosis of exclusion

1.2 Dyspnea

1.2.1 Pulmonary Causes

Possible Diagnosis	Symptoms/Characteristics	Diagnostic Procedures
Pneumothorax	see 1.1 Chest Pain	
Pulmonary embolism	see 1.1 Chest Pain	
Pneumonia	see 1.1 Chest Pain	
COPD exacerbation	• Cough • Poor air movement • Pursed lip breathing • Accessory muscle use for breathing	• Clinical evaluation • Chest Radiography • Arterial Blood Gases (ABGs)
Asthma, bronchospasm, reactive airway disease	• Wheezing, poor air exchange • Arising spontaneously or after stimulus (e.g. cold, exercise, allergen) • Sometimes pulsus paradoxus	• Clinical evaluation • Sometimes pulmonary function testing or bedside peak flow measurement
Foreign body inhalation	• Sudden cough or stridor	• Chest-Radiography (in- and expiratory) • Sometimes bronchoscopy
Obstructive lung disease	• Poor air entry and exit • Barrel chest	• Chest Radiography • Pulmonary function testing
Restrictive lung disease	• Progressive dyspnea	
Interstitial lung disease	• Fine crackles on auscultation	• High-resolution chest CT
Pleural effusion	• Pleuritic chest pain • Lung field that is dull to percussion • Diminished breath sounds	• Chest Radiography-Chest CT • Thoracentesis

1.2.2 Cardiac Causes

Acute myocardial ischemia or MI	see 1.1 Chest Pain	
Papillary muscle dysfunction or rupture	• Sudden onset of chest pain • Holosystolic murmur • Signs of heart failure	• Auscultation • Echocardiography
Heart failure	• Signs of volume overload (peripheral edema, elevated neck veins) • Crackles • S_3 gallop • Dyspnea	• Chest Radiography • ECG • Brain Natriuretic Peptide (BNP) • Echocardiography • Right heart catheterization
Pericardial effusion or tamponade	• Muffled heart sounds • Pulsus paradoxus may be present	• Echocardiography

1.2.3	Other Causes	
Possible Diagnosis	**Symptoms/Characteristics**	**Diagnostic Procedures**
Anxiety disorder, hyperventilation	• Dyspnea often accompanied by psycho-motor agitation • Paresthesias (finger, mouth)	• Normal examination findings • Diagnosis of exclusion
Anemia	• Dyspnea on exertion, progressing to dyspnea at rest	• Complete Blood Count (CBC) • Normal lung examination • Systolic heart murmur may be present

1.3   Syncope

1.3.1	Syncope Because of Arrhythmia	
Bradyarrhythmia	• Syncope occurs without warning • May occur in any position • More common in the elderly	• ECG, if unclear Holter monitor, or event recorder • Electrophysiologic testing • Serum electrolytes
Tachyarrhythmia	• Structural heart disease • Drug intake (e.g. antiarrhythmics) • May occur in any position	
1.3.2	**Syncope Because of Ventricular Dysfunction**	
e. g. acute MI, myocarditis, cardiomyopathy	• Rare symptom of MI, more often in the ederly, with arrythmia or shock	see 1.1 Chest Pain
Pericardial tampo-nade or constriction	• Jugular venous elevation, pulsus para-doxus > 10 mm Hg	• Echocardiography • Sometimes CT
1.3.3	**Syncope Because of Cardiac Flow Obstruction**	
Aortic or mitral stenosis, tetralogy of Fallot, prosthetic valve dehiscence, hypertrophic cardiomyopathy	• Young or old patient, often exertional • Heart murmur	• Echocardiography
Pulmonary embolism	• Usually from large embolus • Tachycardia, dyspnea	• D-dimer • CT angiography or VQ scan

1.3.4   Vasovagal Syncope

Increased thoracic pressure (e.g. Valsalva maneuver, tension pneumothorax, cough), fear, pain, carotid sinus pressure, swallowing	• Warning symptoms (e.g. dizziness, nausea, sweating), prompt but no immediate recovering (5 to 15 min) • Precipitant usually apparent	• Clinical evaluation
Anaphylaxis	• Insect bite, allerigc history, drug intake	• Allergy testing

1.3.5   Orthostatic Syncope

Autonomic dysfunction, drugs (e.g. levodopa, loop diuretics, nitrates, tricyclics)	• Symptoms develop within several minutes of assuming upright position • Drop in Blood Pressure (BP) with standing during examination	• Clinical evaluation • Tilt table testing
Anemia	• Chronic fatigue, sometimes dark stools heavy menses	• CBC

1.3.6   Cerebrovascular Causes of Syncope

Basilar artery transient schemic attack, or stroke	• Ataxia • Sometimes cranial nerve deficits	• CT or MRI
Migraine	• Aura (visual symptoms, photophobia)	• Clinical evaluation

1.3.7   Other Causes of Syncope

Prolonged standing, hyperventilation, hypoglycemia, pregnancy, psychiatric disorders

1.4 Dizziness

1.4.1 Peripheral Vestibular System Disorders

Possible Diagnosis	Symptoms/Characteristics	Diagnostic Procedures
Benign positional vertigo	• Severe brief spinning (trigger: moving head in a specific direction) • Nystagmus	• Dix-Hallpike maneuver (assessment of positional nystagmus) • Hearing and neurologic examination intact
Meniere disease	• Unilateral tinnitus • Hearing loss • Ear fullness (episodes)	• Audiogram • Gadolinum-enhanced MRI
Vestibular neuritis	• Sudden, incapacitating severe vertigo • No hearing loss • No other findings • Lasts up to one week	• Clinical evaluation • Gadolinum-enhanced MRI
Labyrinthitis	• Hearing loss • Tinnitus	• Temporal bone CT • Gadolinum-enhanced MRI
Otitis media	• Ear pain • Discharge (if chronic form) • History of infection	• Clinical evaluation • CT if cholesteatoma (to rule out semicircular canal fistula)
Trauma (e.g. temporal bone fracture, tympanic membrane rupture)	• Trauma obvious on history • Other findings depend on location and extent of damage	• CT
Acoustic neuroma	• Slowly progressive unilateral hearing loss • Tinnitus, dysequilibrium	• CT • MRI
Ototoxic drugs	• Aminoglycoside drugs • Bilateral hearing loss and vestibular loss	• Clinical evaluation
Chronic motion sickness	• Persistent symptoms after acute motion sickness	• Clinical evaluation
Herpes zoster oticus (Ramsay Hunt syndrome)	• Hearing loss often accompanied by facial weakness and loss of taste • Vertigo may be present • Vesicles present on pinna and in ear canal	• Clinical evaluation

1.4.2 Central Vestibular System Disorders

Possible Diagnosis	Symptoms/Characteristics	Diagnostic Procedures
Brain stem hemorrhage or infarction	• Sudden onset • When cochlear artery involved, ear symptoms may occur	• Gadolinum-enhanced MRI or CT • Immediate imaging!
Cerebellar hemorrhage or infarction	• Sudden onset • Ataxia, other cerebellar findings • Headache	
Migraine headache	• Episodic, recurrent vertigo, usually without auditory symptoms • Visual or other auras	• Clinical evaluation • Imaging for exclusion of other diagnosis
Multiple sclerosis	• CNS motor and sensory deficits (remission and recurring exacerbations)	• Gadolinum-enhanced MRI
Vertebral artery dissection	• Head and neck pain	• Magnetic resonance angiography • CT angiography
Vertebrobasilar insufficiency	• Intermittent brief episodes • Sometimes drop attacks • Visual disturbance • Confusion	

1.4.3 Global Disturbances of CNS Function

Anemia	• Blood loss • Iron deficiency	• Complete blood count
CNS drugs (e.g. anticonvulsants, antipsychotics)	• Drugs recently instituted or dose increased, multiple drugs • Elderly patient	
Hypoglycemia	Confusion	Fingerstick glucose test
Hypotension	Symptoms on arising, sometimes with vagal stimulation, but not with head motion or while recumbent	• Orthostatic vital signs, sometimes with tilt table test • Other testing directed at suspected cause
Hypoxemia	• Tachypnea • History of lung disease may be present	• Pulse oximetry

1.4.4 Other Causes

Pregnancy, menstruation, anxiety, depression, thyroid disorders, syphilis

1.5 Palpitations

Symptoms
Perception of cardiac activity (fluttering, racing, or skipping sensation)

Findings	Possible Causes
Occasional skipped beats	• Premature atrial contractions • Premature ventricular contractions
Rapid, regular palpitations with sudden onset and termination	• Paroxysmal supraventricular tachycardia • Atrial flutter with 2:1 atrioventricular (AV) block • Ventricular tachycardia (VT)
Syncope following palpitations	• Sinus node dysfunciton • Wolff-Parkinson-White syndrome • Long QT-syndrome
Palpitations during exercise or an emotional episode	• Healthy person: sinus tachycardia • History of coronary artery disease (CAD): ventricular arrythmia from exercise-induced ischemia
Palpitations following episodic drug use	• Drug intake
Sense of doom, anxiety, or panic	• Suggests (but does not confirm) a psychologic cause
Postoperative patient	• Sinus tachycardia (e.g. infection, pain)
Recurrent episodes since childhood	• Supraventricular arrhythmia (e.g. Wolff-Parkinson-White-syndrome) • Congenital long-QT syndrome
Family history of syncope or sudden death	• Long-QT syndrome • Brugada-syndrome • Inherited cardiomyopathy

1.6 Tachycardia

Possible Diagnosis	Symptoms/Characteristics	Diagnostic Procedures
Supraventricular tachycardia (SVT)	• Palpitations • Dizziness	• ECG
Ventricular tachycardia (VT)	• Palpitations • Dizziness • Chest pain • Syncope	• ECG • Electrophysiologic testing

1.7   Bradycardia

Possible diagnosis	Symptoms/Characteristics	Diagnostic Procedures
Sinus bradycardia	• Lightheadedness • Syncope • Dizziness • Chest pain	• ECG
Heart block	• Syncope • Dizziness • Chest pain • Exercise intolerance	• ECG

1.8   Hypertension/Hypotension

Hypertension	• Headache • Not feeling well, may be asymptomatic	• Clinical evaluation
Hypotension	• Lightheadedness • Dizziness on standing	

1.9   Cyanosis

Cyanosis	• Before the era of pulse oximetry and blood gas analysis, clinicians assessed hypoxemia by looking for cyanosis in the perioral area and fingers. • Approximately 5 g/dL of unoxygenated hemoglobin in the capillaries is required to generate the dark blue color appreciated as cyanosis.	• Pulse oximetry, arterial blood gases

1.10 Edema

Possible Diagnosis	Symptoms/Characteristics	Diagnostic Procedures
Pitting edema	• Pitting edema can be felt by applying pressure to the swollen area with a finger. • The most common systemic diseases associated with edema involve the heart, liver, and kidneys. • In these diseases, edema occurs primarily because of the body's retention of too much sodium and fluid. • Heart failure is a common cause of pitting edema.	• Echocardiogram • Liver function tests • Renal function tests
Non-pitting edema	• Pressure applied to the skin does not result in a persistent indentation. • Non-pitting edema can occur in certain disorders of the lymphatic system such as lymphedema or in thyroid disorders manifesting as pretibial myxedema.	• Clinical evaluation

1.11 Pericardial Effusion

Pericardial effusion	• Pericardial effusion is the presence of an abnormal amount of fluid in the pericardial space. • It can be caused by a variety of local and systemic disorders, or it may be idiopathic. • Pericardial rub, tachycardia, or chest discomfort may be present.	• Chest radiography • Echocardiography
Cardiac tamponade	• Classic triad of pericardial tamponade is presence of hypotension, muffled heart sounds, and jugular venous distension. • Pulsus paradoxus often is present.	• Clinical evaluation • Echocardiography with diastolic RA or RV collapse

1.12   TIA

Possible Diagnosis	Symptoms/Characteristics	Diagnostic Procedures
Transient ischemic attack (TIA)	• A TIA is an acute episode of temporary neurologic dysfunction caused by cerebrovascular occlusion. • Symptoms typically last less than an hour, although they may last up to 24 hours.	• Clinical evaluation • CT or CT angiography • MRI or MR angiography • Carotid duplex studies • Cerebral angiography

1.13   Shock

Hypovolemic shock	• Hypovolemic shock is characterized by rapid fluid or blood loss which results in multiple organ failure due to inadequate circulating volume. • Patients are hypotensive, tachycardic, pale, and ashen in appearance	• CBC, electrolytes, renal function tests • Imaging studies to assess source of blood or fluid loss
Cardiogenic shock	• Cardiogenic shock is characterized by decreased pumping ability of the heart that causes inadequate perfusion to the tissues. The most common cause of cardiogenic shock is large acute myocardial infarction. • Patients are in distress, profoundly diaphoretic, and often have shortness of breath and chest pain.	• ECG • Echocardiogram • Coronary angiography
Septic shock	Septic shock is severe sepsis with persistent hypotension (despite aggressive fluid resuscitation) and resulting tissue hypoperfusion.	• Complete blood count, blood culture • Imaging studies to find source of sepsis

2   Diagnostic Testing

2.1   Murmurs and Heart Sounds

2.1.1   Heart Sounds (abbreviations see page 23)

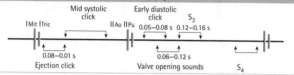

First Heart Sound (S_1)

Caused by the closure of the mitral and tricuspid valves

Loud S_1	Soft S_1
Mitral stenosis	Mitral regurgitation
Short PR interval	Long PR interval
Tachycardia	LBBB, ↑ LVEDP (AS, AI)
Thyrotoxicosis	Immobile mitral valve

Second Heart Sound (S_2)

Caused by the closure of the aortic and pulmonic valves

Wide splitting	Narrow or paradoxical	Fixed
MR, VSD	AS	
RBBB	HCM	
RV volume overload (L→R shunt)	Severe HTN	ASD
RV pressure overload (PS, PAH)	Acute MI, LBBB	

Third Heart Sound (S_3)

- Best heard at the apex with the bell of the stethoscope
- Abnormal for age > 40 yrs
- Suggests an enlarged ventricular chamber
- Associated with: MR, TR, and CHF

Fourth Heart Sound (S_4)

- Best heard at the apex with the bell of the stethoscope
- Suggests decreased ventricular compliance
- Associated with: LVH, HTN, AS, HCM, PAH, MI, acute MR, and PS

2.1.2   Murmurs

Innocent vs. Pathologic Murmurs	
Innocent murmurs	Pathologic murmurs
Peak or end in the first half of systole	Diastolic murmur
Less than III/IV in intensity	New or very loud > III/IV
Loudest at LLSB without radiation	Abnormally split S_2
Intensity decreases with Valsalva maneuver	Intensity increases with Valsalva maneuver
Patient younger than 45 yrs	Patient older than 45 yrs

Murmurs: Differential Diagnoses

Systolic	AS, PS, high flow states (anemia, pregnancy, adolescence), ASD, MVP, HCM
Holosystolic	MR, TR, VSD
Diastolic	AR, PR, MS, TS, ASD
Continuous	PDA, coarctation of aorta, AV fistula, mammary souffle (in pregnancy)

Grading of Murmurs

Grade	Description
1	Very faint
2	Soft
3	Heard all over the precordium
4	Loud, with palpable thrill (i.e. a tremor or vibration felt on palpation)
5	Very loud, with thrill. May be heard when stethoscope is partly off the chest.
6	Very loud, with thrill. May be heard with stethoscope entirely off the chest

Abbreviations

AI	Aortic insufficiency	MS	Mitral stenosis
AR	Aortic regurgitation	MVP	Mitral valve prolapse
AS	Aortic stenosis	PAH	Pulmonary arterial hypertension
ASD	Atrial septal defect	PDA	Patent ductus arteriosus
CHF	Congestive heart failure	PR	Pulmonary regurgitation, PR interval
HCM	Hypertrophic cardiomyopathy	PS	Pulmonary stenosis
HTN	Hypertension	RBBB	Right bundle branch block
LBBB	Left bundle branch block	RV	Right ventricle, right ventricular
LVEDP	Left ventricular end-diastolic pressure	TR	Tricuspid regurgitation
MI	Myocardial infarction	TS	Tricuspid stenosis
MR	Mitral regurgitation, magnetic resonance	VSD	Ventricular septal defect

2.2   Chest Radiography

2.2.1   Standard Chest Radiograph: Posterior-Anterior and Lateral Views

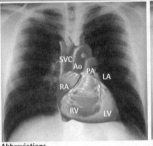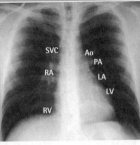

Abbreviations

SVC: Superior vena cava
PA: Pulmonary artery
RA: Right atrium
LA: Left atrium

RV: Right ventricle
LV: Left ventricle
Ao = Aorta

Description	• Radiograph of the chest, typically used to diagnose conditions affecting the heart, lung, and mediastinum. • The procedure of obtaining a chest radiograph employs ionizing radiation in the form of X-rays to generate images. The typical radiation dose to an adult from a chest radiograph is approximately 0.02-0.05 mSv.
Different views from the chest	• By changing the relative orientation of the body and the direction of the X-ray beams, different views are obtained • The most commonly performed views are the posteroanterior (PA), antero-posterior (AP), and lateral views. • Typical views used are the PA and lateral views, with the AP view used mostly for portable bedside imaging.
PA view	The X-ray source is positioned so that X-rays enter through the posterior aspect of the chest, and exit out of the anterior aspect where they are detected.
AP view	Positions of the X-ray source and detector are reversed: X-rays enter through the anterior aspect and exit through the posterior aspect of the chest
Lateral view	Obtained in a similar fashion as the PA/AP views, except that in the lateral view, the patient stands with both arms raised and the left side of the chest is pressed against a flat surface.

Indications	Chest radiographs are commonly used to provide evaluation of cardiac patients with chest symptoms and signs and to confirm diagnosis. These include:
	• **Symptom evaluation:**
	- Chest pain - Orthopnea or paroxysmal nocturnal
	- Shortness of breath dyspnea
	• **Confirm or recognize need for additional imaging:**
	- Heart failure - Suspected aortic dissection
	• **Assess position:**
	- Central venous catheters - Intra-aortic Balloon Pumps (IABP)
	- Pacemakers/ICDs - Prosthetic heart valves

2.2.2   Typical Findings in Cardiac Conditions

Heart failure	• Cardiomegaly • Pleural effusion • Fluid in the major fissure	• Horizontal lines in the periphery of lower posterior lung fields (Kerley B lines).
Pulmonary embolism	• Often normal • May reveal subtle changes in the blood vessel patterns and signs of pulmonary infarction	
Aortic dissection	• Widened mediastinum • Calcium sign is the separation of the intimal calcification from the outer aortic soft tissue border by 10 mm	• Pleural effusions • Obliteration of the aortic knob • Depression of the left mainstem bronchus • Chest radiograph is normal in approximately 10% to12% of patients with aortic dissection
Constrictive pericarditis	• Lateral chest radiographs often show pericardial calcification	

2.2.3   Contraindications

- There are no absolute contraindications to chest radiography.
- Radiation exposure is relatively contraindicated in children and pregnant women, and clinicians should weigh the benefits of obtaining the study against the risk of radiation exposure

2.3 ECG

2.3.1 ECG Evaluation

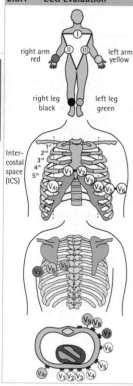

right arm
red

left arm
yellow

right leg
black

left leg
green

Intercostal space (ICS)

1st
2nd
3rd
4th
5th

Cross section of the heart (V_1 to V_9)

1. Einthoven's extremity (limb) leads (I, II, III)

Bipolar leads. The amplitude is positive if the depolarization moves towards the positive electrode marked with ⊕.

| right arm: red cable |
| left arm: yellow cable |
| left leg: green cable |
| **right leg: black ground cable** |

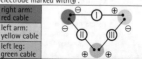

2. Wilson's chest (precordial) leads (V_1 to V_6)

Unipolar leads. They measure the voltage of any one electrode relative to a constructed zero potential.

V_1	4th ICS at the right sternal border
V_2	4th ICS at the left sternal border
V_3	midway between V_2 and V_4
V_4	5th ICS at the midclavicular line
V_5	5th ICS at the left anterior axillary line
V_6	5th ICS at the left midaxillary line

3. Additional Wilson's leads (V_7 to V_9)

Unipolar leads. They measure electrocardiographic changes on the inferior cardiac wall. Limb cables (red, yellow, green) as well as V_1 to V_3 or V_4 to V_6 could be attached.

V_7	5th ICS at the left posterior axillary line
V_8	5th ICS at the midscapulary line
V_9	5th ICS at the left paravertebral line
right leg: black ground cable	

Cross section of the heart (V_1 to V_9)

If a right ventricular infarction is suspected, V_{4r} on the right side of the chest is useful.

Caution: Placing the electrodes improperly, for example, in the second intercostal space, may lead to an R reduction in the anterior leads and may, therefore, be misinterpreted as an old anterior myocardial infarction.

2.3.2   ECG Interpretation

Normal Values

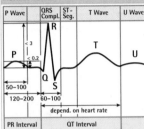

P Wave	QRS Compl.	ST-Seg.	T Wave	U Wave

Periods in ms, amplitudes in mV

Heart Rate/min	PR Interval (s)	QT Interval (s)
60	max. 0.2	0.35–0.43
70	max. 0.19	0.32–0.40
80	max. 0.18	0.30–0.37
90	max. 0.17	0.29–0.35
100	max. 0.16	0.27–0.33

Axis Deviation

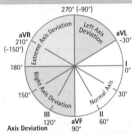

Clinical Examples of Axis Deviations

-30° to -90° is left axis deviation:
Inferior wall MI, left anterior hemiblock

+120° to 180° is right axis deviat. (RAD):
Left posterior hemi-block, right ventricular hypertrophy, lateral wall infarct, lead reversal, dextrocardia

>180° is extreme right axis: same dd as RAD

2.3.3   Normal ECG Findings

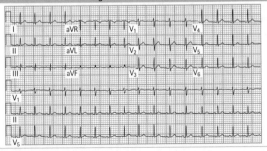

2.3.4   Pathologic ECG Findings

Hypertrophy

Right atrial enlargement	Elevated, peaked P wave > 0.2 mV, particularly in II, III and aVF.	
Left atrial enlargement	Widening of P wave > 0.1 s, particular in I, II and V_1–V_3. In V_1 often biphasic P with a marked negative deflection.	
Right ventricular hypertrophy	R V_2 + S V_5 > 10.5 mm; right axis deviation, sometimes RBBBlike ECG	
Left ventricular hypertrophy	Sokolow index: S V_2 + R V_5 > 35 mm; left axis deviation	

Bundle Branch Blocks

Left anterior fascicular block	No widening of the QRS, but left axis deviation.
Right anterior fascicular block	No widening of the QRS, but right axis deviation.
Incompl. LBBB	Widening of the QRS > 0.10 s, but < 0.12 s
Complete LBBB	Widening of the QRS > 0.12 s, delay of terminal negativity in V_6 > 0.05 s, frequent loss of R on ant. wall, left precordial repolarization disturbance and ST-elevation.
Complete RBBB	Widening of the QRS > 0.12 s, delay of terminal negativity in V_1 > 0.03 s, frequent rSr' compl. in V_1, repolarization disturbance in V_1–V_3.

Pathologic ECG Findings

AV Conduction Defects

First degree AV Block	Consistent delay in conduction, PR interval > 0.20 s.	 AV-Block I°
Second degree AV Block, Mobitz Type I	Intermittent conduction failure with missing QRS complexes, progressive prolongation of PR intervals until a P wave is blocked.	 AV-Block II° (Type Wenckebach)
Second degree AV Block, Mobitz Type II	Intermittent failure of the AV conduction, the PR interval remains within normal limits.	 AV-Block II° (Type Mobitz)
Third degree AV Block (Total Block)	Complete conduction block of all electrical impulses between atria and ventricles, atria and ventricles beat independently.	 AV-Block III°

Carditis, Cardiomyopathy

Acute pericarditis	Simultaneous ST elevations on the anterior and posterior wall, typically originating from the S wave, can be misinterpreted as MI.	 Acute pericarditis
Hypertrophic (obstructive) cardiomyopathy	Signs of left ventricular hypertrophy (Sokolow index), varying ST segment changes without classic localization and deep, inverted T waves.	
Dilated cardiomyopathy	Nonspecific repolarization disturbances	

Bradyarrhythmias

Junctional escape rhythms	**1. Upper Junctional Rhythm:** P waves in I, II, III, aVF are neg., PR Interval can be short. **2. Central Junction. Rhythm:** P waves are hidden in the QRS. **3. Lower Junctional Rhythm:** P waves are negative in I, II, III and located after the QRS complex
First degree Sinoatrial (SA) Block	Prolongation of sinoatrial conduction time. Not visible on ECG.

Second degree SA Block, Wenckebach	Progressive prolongation of the SA conduction with an ultimate interruption in conduction. Sinus intervals shorten until a break occurs which is shorter than two PP intervals.	SA-Block II° (Type Wenckebach)
Second degree SA Block, Mobitz	Intermittent sinus pauses that are a multiple of the sinus interval.	SA-Block II° (Type Mobitz)
Third degree SA Block	Complete block. Escape rhythm from a junction or ventricular depolarization site.	

Reflex Bradycardia

Carotid sinus syndrome	Pressure on the carotid sinus can cause sinus bradycardia and AV block, sometimes with vasodilatation and hypotension.
Neurocardiogenic syncope	Stimulation of mechanoreceptors (left ventricular) results in bradycardia and peripheral vasodilatation leading to hypotension.

Electrolyte Disturbances, Drugs

Hypokalemia	Repolarization disorders, ST depression, prominent U wave, may merge into TU waves.	Hypokalemia
Hyperkalemia	Tall, peaked T waves that later flatten, broad QRS complex. Finally, tachycardic arrhythmias can occur resulting in bradycardia and asystole.	Hyperkalemia
Hypercalcemia	Shortening of the corrected QT Interval (QTc).	Hypercalcemia ▬ = QT shortened
Hypocalcemia	Prolongation of the QT Interval.	Hypocalcemia ▬ =QT prolonged
ECG changes induced by Digitalis	Shallow ST depressions. AV blocks possible.	Digitalis effect

2.3.5   Myocardial Ischemia

Angina	Horizontal or descending ST depression		
Myocardial infarction, early stage	Tall T wave	A few minutes after onset	
Myocardial infarction, stage I	ST elevation and R waves are present, no Q waves, T waves are still positive	Up to 6 h	
Myocardial infarction, intermediate stage	ST elevation and R wave decrease, Q waves arise and inverted T waves appear.	> 6 hours	
Myocardial infarction, next stage	Q waves develop, R wave will disappear.	Days	
Myocardial infarction, stage III	Loss of R wave in the leads. Q waves may be found, T wave becomes pos. again and ST elevat. disappears.	Residual	
Non-Q-wave MI	Subdendocardial infarction of the anterior wall with T wave inversion over anterior precordial leads, no ST elevations, no R loss, no Q waves.		

Infarct Localization

	I	II	III	aVL	aVF	rV4	V2	V3	V4	V5	V6
Apical	+			+			+	+	+		
Anteroseptal							+	+			
Anterolateral	+			+						+	+
Posterolateral			+		+					+	+
Inferior		+	+		+						
Right ventricular			+		+	+	(+)				

2.4   Exercise Stress Test

Definition	• Reliable and widely used method of evaluating patients who have or are at risk of developing cardiovascular disease. • In addition to the data from ECG changes (ST segment, T-and U-wave abnormalities), other significant data such as arrhythmias, heart rate, blood pressure, exercise capacity, and rating of perceived exertion can be derived from the test to aid in patient evaluation and treatment. • Exercise testing is typically performed using either an electrically driven treadmill or, less often, a bicycle with exercise protocols that are individualized based on the patient's baseline exertional capacity. • The test includes continuous ECG monitoring for the presence of arrhythmias and ischemic ECG changes during exercise and recovery, and blood pressure monitoring at each stage of exercise.
Indications	• Patients undergoing initial evaluation with suspected or known CAD • Patients with suspected or known CAD, previously evaluated, now presenting with significant change in clinical status • Low-risk patients with unstable angina, eight to 12 hours after presentation, who have been free of active symptoms of ischemia or heart failure • Intermediate-risk patients with unstable angina, two to three days after presentation, who have been free of active symptoms of ischemia or heart failure • Intermediate-risk patients with unstable angina who have initial cardiac markers that are normal, repeat electrocardiography without significant change, and cardiac markers that are normal, 6 to 12 hours after the onset of symptoms, and no other evidence of ischemia during observation • In patients with acute myocardial infarction before discharge for prognostic assessment, activity prescription or evaluation of medical therapy (submaximal stress test at four to six days) • In chronic aortic regurgitation, assessment of functional capacity and symptomatic responses in patients with a history of equivocal symptoms
Method	• Treadmill or bicycle exercise to 85% of age-predicted maximum heart rate (220 minus age (years)) with continuous ECG monitoring (ie, exercise ECG). • The test may be done in conjunction with an imaging modality such as echocardiography or nuclear imaging • Pharmacologic stress testing should be considered when patients are unable to exercise.
ECG interpretation	• A positive stress test is defined as having ≥1 mm ST-segment depression. • ST-depression only in inferior leads provides little localization value. • ST-elevation occurs in approximately 0.1% of patients and localizes the ischemic area (nondiagnostic if pre-existing Q waves).

Correlates of Ischemia in the Exercise ECG

| J-Point | ST-Depression | ST-Depression | ST-Depression |
| 80 ms | | | |

When to Stop the Stress Test

Absolute end points	• Systolic blood pressure drop of >10 mm Hg from baseline, when associated with other evidence of ischemia • Moderate to severe angina • Nervous system symptoms ↑ (i.e., near-syncope, ataxia, light-headedness, vertigo) • Patient's desire to terminate exercise • Sustained ventricular tachycardia • ST-elevation of 1 mm in leads without pathologic Q-waves
Relative endpoints	• Systolic blood pressure drop of >10 mm Hg from baseline in the absence of other evidence of ischemia • ECG changes such as > 2 mm ST depressions or marked axis shift • Arrhythmias other than sustained ventricular tachycardia (supraventricular tachycardia, bradyarrhythmias, heart block, multifocal PVCs, triplets of PVCs) • Fatigue, shortness of breath, wheezing, leg cramps, or claudication • Bundle branch block that cannot be distinguished from ventric. tachycardia • Increasing chest pain • Hypertensive response to exercise, defined as systolic blood pressure > 250 mm Hg, diastolic blood pressure >115 mm Hg, or both

Contraindications

Absolute	• Acute myocardial infarction within 48 hours • Unstable angina not previously stabilized by medical therapy • Uncontrolled cardiac arrhythmias causing symptoms or hemodyn. compromise • Symptomatic severe aortic stenosis • Uncontrolled symptomatic heart failure • Acute pulmonary embolus or pulmonary infarction • Acute myocarditis or pericarditis, acute aortic dissection
Relative	• Moderate stenotic valvular heart disease • Severe arterial hypertension • Tachyarrhythmias or bradyarrhythmias • Hypertrophic cardiomyopathy and other forms of outflow tract obstruction • Physical impairment leading to inability to exercise adequately • High degree atrioventricular block

Role of Stress Testing in Stable Angina

For patients with suspected stable angina, stress testing is most useful for those with an intermediate pretest probability of CAD; the pretest probability can be determined by assessing the type of chest pain and the age and sex of the patient.

1. Assess Chest Pain Type

Typical angina	1. Presence of pressure or pain in a classic location and of normal duration
	2. Pain is provoked by exertion or emotional stress
	3. Pain is relieved by rest or nitroglycerin
Atypical angina	Presence of any 2 of the above features
Nonanginal pain	Presence of 1 or none of the above features

Reprinted from the Journal of the American College of Cardiology, 1 (2), Diamond GA, A Clinically Relevant Classification of Chest Discomfort, 574-5. Copyright 1983, with permission from the American College of Cardiology Foundation. Published by Elsevier Inc.

2. Determine the Pretest Probability of CAD

Age (y)	Sex	Typical angina	Atypical angina	Nonanginal pain	Asymptomatic
30–39	M	Intermediate	Intermediate	Low	Very low
	F	Intermediate	Very low	Very low	Very low
40–49	M	High	Intermediate	Intermediate	Low
	F	Intermediate	Low	Very low	Very low
50–59	M	High	Intermediate	Intermediate	Low
	F	Intermediate	Intermediate	Low	Very low
60–69	M	High	Intermediate	Intermediate	Low
	F	High	Intermediate	Intermediate	Low

Probabilities: High: > 90%; intermediate: 10%–90%; low: < 10%; very low: < 5%.

Reprinted from the Journal of the American College of Cardiology, 30 (1), Gibbons RJ, et al., ACC/AHA Guidelines for Exercise Testing. A Report of the American College of Cardiology/American Heart Association Task Force on Practice Guidelines (Committee on Exercise Testing), 260-315,. Copyright 1997, with permission from the American College of Cardiology and the American Heart Association Inc. Published by Elsevier Science Inc.

3. Stress Test is Most Useful in Patients With an Intermediate Probability of CAD

Low CAD probability	Intermediate CAD probability	High CAD probability
High false positive rate	Optimal	High false negative rate

Further Risk Stratification

Use the Duke-Treadmill Score which provides useful prognostic information (see →75). The Duke-Treadmill Score is based on the Bruce protocol

The Bruce Protocol*

- The most widely used treadmill exercise protocol; this allows for a great amount of normative data and, therefore, comparison.
- Major disadvantage: large increments of change in workload between stages can be difficult for less fit individuals.

Stage	Minutes	Grade (%)	Speed (miles per hour)	
1	3	10	1.7	4.7
2	6	12	2.5	7
3	9	14	3.4	10.1
4	12	16	4.2	12.9
5	15	18	5.0	15.0

*The modified Bruce protocol has been developed for less fit individuals and adds stages 0 and 0.5, which are performed at 1.7 mph and a 0% grade, increasing to a 5% grade. This provides a lower workload for patients with poor cardiovascular fitness. Other protocols have been developed, such as the Naughton protocol, which has a more gradual increase in workload, and the Balke protocol, which maintains a steady speed and increases the grade every 2 minutes. The exercise protocol should be selected to suit the individual patient.

Other Markers of Worse Prognosis

- Failure to achieve 5 METs (metabolic equivalent)
- ST segment changes within the first 2 stages of Bruce protocol
- Inability to achieve target heart rate (chronotropic incompetence)
- Abnormal heart rate recovery (change in heart rate of ≤ 12 beats per minute from maximum exercise heart rate at 2 min)
- Drop in systolic blood pressure during exercise
- Chest pain during test

Key Point

As exercise time and METs achieved are important determinants for prognosis, patients should exercise beyond target heart rate to maximal capacity, if possible.

2.4.1   Pharmacologic Stress Testing

Used substances are adenosine, regadenoson, dipyridamole, dobutamine

Adenosine (vasodilator)

Mechanism	• Causes coronary artery vasodilatation via up-regulation of cAMP production.
	• Vasodilation helps to detect coronary stenosis by causing a discrepancy in blood flow, because diseased coronary arteries are already max. dilated and therefore have a diminished vasodilat. response to adenosine compared to healthy vessels.
	• In the presence of stenosis, a coronary steal phenomenon can occur in which blood flow is diverted from diseased to healthy vessels, thereby causing ischemia.

Contra-indications	Asthma, emphysema	Adenosine can cause bronchospasm; pat. with asthma or emphysema have a relative contraindication for adenosine stress testing.
	AV-block	Because adenosine can cause transient AV block, pat. with 2nd degree AV block or higher should not undergo adenosine testing.

Key points	• Patients who are on β-blockers and other negative chronotropes can safely and accurately undergo adenosine stress testing.
	• Caffeine is a competitive adenosine-inhibitor (refrain ingestion 24 h prior testing)
	• Chest pain during infusion is frequent but not very clinically significant.
	• ECG changes during infusion are infrequent, although clinically significant.

Regadenoson (A$_2$A adenosine receptor agonist)

Mechanism	Acts as a coronary vasodilator; may be used as an alternative pharmacologic stressor.
Key points	• Delivered as a rapid intravenous injection, which increases its ease of use in comparison with adenosine which requires infusion.
	• A2A adenosine receptor selectivity leads to lower incidence of adenosine-related adverse effects of AV block and bronchoconstriction.

Dipyridamole (indirect coronary vasodilator)

Mechanism	Works by increasing intravascular adenosine levels via inhibition of deamination (the mechanism of inducing a perfusion abnormality is similar to that of adenosine, with coronary steal occurring more frequently)
Key points	May be reversed with aminophylline; Indications and contraind. similar to adenosine

Dobutamine

Mechanism	A synthetic catecholamine and acts as a β1- and a β2-agonist, resulting in increased heart rate, blood pressure, and myocardial contractility. This mimics the physiologic response to exercise and produces perfusion abnormalities by the development of regional ischemia.
Key points	• May be reversed with esmolol.
	• Should be considered in patients who cannot exercise and have a contraindication to vasodilator pharmacologic stress testing.
	• Contraindicated in patients with recent MI, unstable angina, significant aortic stenosis, HOCM, or a history of tachyarrhythmia.

Stress-Echocardiography Protocol

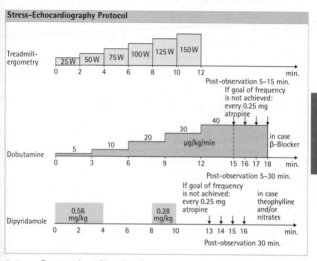

2.5   Pacemaker Checking

General

- Pacemakers must be checked periodically to make sure that they are functioning correctly.
- Some testing can actually be done over the phone, using a process called **transtelephonic monitoring**.
- More detailed testing of the pacemaker should be done in person (may be performed twice in the first 6 months after pacemaker insertion and then every 6 months thereafter)
- Checking the pacemaker at periodic intervals is important because the battery wears down over time and there is a small risk that one of the electrical leads implanted in the heart can dislodge, fracture, or malfunction.

Components of Pacemaker Clinic Visit Check

- Skin overlying the pacemaker system
- > 12 sec multi-channel ECG rhythm recording with and without magnet application over the generator
- Lead stability testing, respiratory tests and lead integrity by generator manipulation
- End-of-life check - use of a device specific programmer is mandatory
- Verification of pacing and sensing functions by threshold assessment using the programmer and/or (where appropriate and applicable) magnet application
- Recording and communicating all the above as appropriate

Transtelephonic Monitoring (TTM)

Goals of TTM non-magnet ECG assessment	• Determine whether the patient displays intrinsic rhythm or is being intermittently or continuously paced at the programmed settings. • Characterize the patient's underlying atrial mechanism; for example, sinus versus atrial fibrillation, atrial tachycardia, etc. • If intrinsic rhythm is displayed, determine that normal (appropriate) sensing is present for 1 or both chambers depending on whether it is a single- or dual-chamber pacemaker and programmed pacing mode.
Goals of TTM ECG assessment during magnet application	• Verify effective capture of the appropriate chamber(s) depending on whether it is a single- or dual-chamber pacemaker, and verify the programmed pacing mode. • Assess magnet rate. Once magnet rate is determined, it should be compared with values obtained on previous transmissions to determine whether any change has occurred. • The person assessing the TTM also should be aware of the magnet rate that represents elective replacement indicators for that pacemaker. • If the pacemaker is one in which pulse width is 1 of the elective replacement indicators, the pulse width should also be assessed and compared with previous values. • If the pacemaker has some mechanism to allow transtelephonic assessment of threshold (i.e., Threshold Margin Test [TMTTM]) and that function is programmed "on," the results of this test should be demonstrated and analyzed. • If a dual-chamber pacemaker is being assessed and magnet application results in a change in AV interval during magnet application, that change should be demonstrated and verified.

2.6 Echocardiography

General	• In echocardiography, sound is directed into the body and reflected by interfaces between tissues of different acoustic impedance, such as myocardium, valves and blood.
	• Two dimensional (2D) echocardiography uses the principle of ultrasound reflection off cardiac structures to produce images of the heart and is an ideal imaging modality for assessing left ventricular (LV) size, function and valves.
	• Doppler echocardiography is a method for detecting the direction and velocity of moving blood within the heart.
	• Doppler methods extend the use of cardiac ultrasonography to the evaluation of normal and abnormal flow states and provide quantitative data for patients with heart diseases.

See abbreviations on page 43

Aortic Stenosis (AS)

	Peak Velocity	Peak Grad.
Normal	1.0 m/s	< 10 mm Hg
Mild	< 3.0 m/s	< 20 mm Hg
Moderate	3.0–4.4 m/s	20–64 mm Hg
Severe	> 4.5 m/s	> 64 mm Hg

Mitral Stenosis (MS)

	Mean Grad.	End Diast. Grad.	Area
Normal	–	0–2 mm Hg	4–6 cm²
Mild	≤ 5 mm Hg	2–6 mm Hg	1.5–2.5 cm²
Moderate	6–15 mm Hg	7–12 mm Hg	1.1–1.5 cm²
Severe	> 15 mm Hg	> 12 mm Hg	< 1.0 cm²

MV Pressure Half Time in MS

Normal	30–60 ms
Abnormal	90–400 ms
Gray area	60–90 ms
Mild	90–150 ms
Moderate	150–219 ms
Severe	≥ 220 ms

Criteria for Diagnosis of Significant MS

MV orifice area	< 1 cm
Mean pressure gradient	> 10 mm Hg
Pressure half-time	> 220 ms
PA systolic pressure	> 35 mm Hg

MS Morphology Scoring (Score)

Mobility	Pts	Subvalvular Apparatus	Pts
Highly mobile with restricted leaflet tips	1	Min. thickening below the mitral leaflets	1
Leaflet middle and base with normal mobility	2	Thickening of chordal structures extending into 1/3 of the chordal length	2
Valve continues to move forward in diastole, mainly from the base	3	Thickening extending to the distal third of chordal length	3
No or minimal forward movement of leaflet in diastole	4	Extensive thickening and shortening of all chordal structures	4

Pts. = points

Thickening	Pts	Calcification	Pts
Near normal thickness (4–5mm)	1	A single area of ↑ echo brightness	1
Mid leaflet normal, marked thickening in margins (5–8mm)	2	Scattered areas of brightness confined to leaflet margins	2
Thickening extending through entire leaflet (5–8mm)	3	Brightness extending into the mid portion of the leaflets	3
Marked thickening of all leaflet tissue (8–10mm)	4	Extensive brightness throughout much of the leaflet tissue	4

Score ≤ 8 = MS appropriate for valvuloplasty; Score > 8 = MS not appropriate for valvuloplasty

Pulmonic Stenosis (PS)

	Peak Gradient	Valve Area
Mild	5–30 mm Hg	> 1.0 cm²
Moderate	30–64 mm Hg	0.5–1.0 cm²
Severe	> 64 mm Hg	< 0.5 cm²

Tricuspid Stenosis (TS)

	Mean Grad.	Valve Area
Normal	–	7–9 cm²
Mild	< 2 mm Hg	–
Moderate	2–6 mm Hg	–
Severe	> 7 mm Hg	< 2 cm²

Valvular Regurgitation

Valve	Normal Peak Velocity
Aortic	3–5 m/s
Mitral	4–6 m/s
Pulmonic	≥ 1.5 m/s
Tricuspid	2.5 m/s

Aortic Regurgitation

	Deceleration Rate	Press Half Time
Mild	< 2 m/s²	≥ 500 ms
Moderate	2–3 m/s²	350–500 ms
Mod. Severe	–	200–350 ms
Severe	> 3 m/s²	≤ 200 ms

Mitral Regurgitation (MR)

	Jet Area	Vena Contracta
Mild	< 4cm² or < 20% LA	< 0.3 cm
Mild-Mod.	4–6cm² or 20-30% LA	≥ 0.7 cm
Mod.-Sev.	6–8cm² or 30-40% LA	≥ 0.7 cm
Severe	≥8–10cm² or > 40% LA	≥ 0.7 cm

	Regurg Vol	RF(%)	ROA
Mild	< 30	< 30	< 0.20 cm²
Mild-Mod.	30–44	30–39	0.2–0.29 cm²
Mod.-Sev.	45–59	40–49	0.3–0.39 cm²
Severe	≥ 60	≥ 50	≥ 0.40 cm²

Mitral Valve Scallops

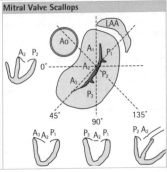

Normal Doppler Data for Prosthetic Aortic Valves

Valve Type	Size (mm)	Vmax (m/s)	Mean Grad (mmHg)	V Ratio	AVA (cm²)
Mechanical Valves					
Bi-leaflet (St. Jude)	19	3.0 (2.0–4.5)	20 (10–30)	0.37	1.0
	21	2.7 (2.5–3.5)	14 (10–30)	0.40	1.3
	23	2.5 (2.0–3.5)	12 (10–30)	0.37	1.3
	25	2.4 (2.0–3.5)	12 (5–30)	0.42	1.8
	27	2.2 (2.0–3.1)	11 (5–20)	0.46	2.4
	29	2.0 (2.0–2.5)	10 (5–15)	0.49	2.7
	31	2.1 (1.5–2.5)	10 (5–15)	0.49	3.1
Tilting-disk (Bjork-Shiley, Medtronic Hall)	19	2.1±0.7			
	21	2.8±0.9	16		
	23	2.6±0.4	14±5		
	25	2.1±0.3	13±3		
	27	1.9±0.2	10±3		
	29	1.9±0.2	7±6		
Ball-cage (Starr-Edwards)		3.1±0.5	24±4		
Tissue Valves					
Stented porcine tissue (Hancock or Carpentier-Edwards)	19	2.8±0.7	16±2		15±0.1
	21	2.6±0.4	15±6		1.8±0.2
	23	2.6±0.4	13±6		2.1±0.2
	25	2.5±0.4	11±2		
	27	2.4±0.4	10±1		
	29	2.4±0.4	12		
Pericardial valve (CE Perimount)		1.5±0.9			2.5±0.6
Mosaic valve (Medtronic) 23mm		2.3±1.2			
SPV (St. Jude)		2.2±0.4			1.8–2.3
Aortic homograft		1.8±0.4			2.2 (1.7–3.1)

Normal Doppler Data for Prosthetic Mitral Valves				
Valve Type	Vmax (m/s)	Mean Grad (mm Hg)	T1/2 (mm/s)	MVA (cm²)
Mechanical				
Bi-leaflet (St Jude)	1.6±0.3	4±1	77±17	2.9±0.6
Tilting-disk (Bjork-Shiley)	1.6±0.3	3±2	90±22	2.4±0.6
Ball-cage (Starr-Edwards)	1.9±0.5	5±2	110±27	2.0±0.5
Porcine Tissue				
Ionescu-Shiley	1.5±0.3	3±1	93±25	2.4±0.8
Carpentier-Edwards	1.8±0.2	6±2	85±25	2.5±0.7

Important Formulas	
AVA (Cont Eq)	$A_2 = A_1 \times TVI_1/TVI_2$
Pressure gradient	$4(v)^2$
RVSP	$[4(v)^2 + \text{Est. RA P}]$
LA pressure	$SBP - 4(MR\ V_{max})^2$
Q_p	$CSA_{PA} \times TVI_{PA}$
Q_s	$CSA_{LVOT} \times TVI_{LVOT}$
PISA	$2\pi r^2$
RV	PISA x $V_{aliasing}$
RV	ROA x VTI_{MR}
MVA	220/PHT

	M-Mode (cm)	2-D Measurement (cm)
RVID d	0.9 – 2.6	1.9 – 3.8
RVID s	1.5 – 2.2	–
IVS d	0.6 – 1.1	0.6 – 1.1
IVS s	0.9 – 1.8	–
LVID d	3.7 – 5.6	3.5 – 6.0
LVID s	2.0 – 4.0	2.1 – 4.0
LPW d	0.6 – 1.1	0.6 – 1.1
LPW s	0.9 – 1.8	–
LA diam	2.0 – 4.0	< 5.5
Ao root diam	2.0 – 3.7	–
Ao cusp sep	1.5 – 2.6	–

Normal Valve Area (cm²)	
AV area	3 – 5
MV area	3.5 – 5.5
TV area	7 – 9

Normal Reference Values	
LVOT	1.8 – 2.2 cm
Fractional shortening	28 – 41 % (33 %)
EF	45 – 90 % (62 %)
IVS% thickening	27 – 70 % (46 %)
LPW thickening	25 – 80 % (45 %)
VTI MV	10 – 13 cm
LVOT	18 – 22 cm
Aorta	12.6 – 22.5 cm
D/E excursion	1.8 – 2.8 cm
E/F slope	70 – 150 mm/s
EPSS	2 – 12 mm
AO annulus	1.4 – 2.6 cm
Asc aorta	2.1 – 3.4 cm
MV annulus	2.3 ± 0.5 cm
Sinus of Valsalva	2.1 – 3.5 cm

Normal Valve Velocities		
Valve	Peak Velocity	Range (m/s)
AV	1.3 m/s	0.1 – 1.7
LVOT	0.9 m/s	0.7 – 1.1
MV	0.9 m/s	0.6 – 1.3
PV/art	0.75 m/s	0.6 – 0.9
TV	0.5 m/s	0.3 – 0.7

TEE – Atheroma Grading	
Grade I	Normal to mild intimal thickening
Grade II	Severe intimal thickening without protruding atheroma
Grade III	Atheroma protruding < 5 mm
Grade IV	Atheroma protruding > 5 mm
Grade V	Atheroma of any size with mobile components

Abbreviations

A_1	Lateral scallop of anterior mitral leaflet	MVA	Mitral valve area
A_2	Central scallop of anterior mitral leaflet	PISA	Proximal isovelocity surface area
Ao	Aortic valve	PV	Pulmonary valve
AV	Aortic valve velocity	Q_p	Pulmonary flow
AVA	Aortic valve area	Q_s	Systemic flow
CSA_{LVOT}	Cross sectional area left ventricular outflow tract	RA	Right atrium
		ROA	Regurgitant orifice area
CSA_{PA}	Cross sectional area pulmonary artery	RV	Right ventricle
EF	Ejection fraction	RVA	Right ventricular apex
EPSS	E point to septal separation	RVID	Right ventricular internal diameter
IVS_d	Interventricular septal thickness (diast.)	RV	Regurgitant volume
IVS_s	Interventricular septal thickness (syst.)	RVSP	Right ventricular systolic pressure
LPW	Left ventricular posterior wall	SBP	Systolic blood pressure
LVID	Left ventricular internal diameter	TV	Tricuspid Valve
MV	Mitral valve	VTI	Velocity time integral

LA Volume and Pressure Assessment

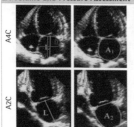

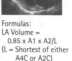

Formulas:
LA Volume =
0.85 x A1 x A2/L
(L = Shortest of either A4C or A2C)
LA Volume =
(D1 x D2 x D3) x 0.523
LA Pressure =
E/Em + 4

LA Volume/BSA (ml/m²)	
Normal	22±6
Mild increase	29-33
Moderate incr.	34-39
Severe increase	≥ 40

LA Pressure (mm Hg)	
Normal	6-12
Decr. relaxation	8-14
Pseudonormal	15-22
Restrictive	>22

Tamponade vs. Pericarditis vs. Cardiomyopathy			
	Pericardial Tamponade	Constrictive Pericarditis	Restrictive Cardiomyopathy
Hemodynamics			
RA pressure	↑	↑	↑
RV/LV filling pressure	↑, RV = LV	↑, RV = LV	↑, LV > RV
PA pressure	Normal	Mild ↑ (35 – 40 mmHg)	Mod – Severe ↑ (= 60 mmHg)
RV diastolic pressure plateau		> 1/3 peak RV pressure	< 1/3 peak RV pressure
Radionuclide diastolic filling		Rapid early filling Impaired late filling	Impaired early filling
2D Echo	Moderate to large effusion	Pericardial thickening without effusion	LVH Normal systolic function
Doppler Echo	Reciprocal respiratory changes in RV and LV filling	E > a on LV inflow Prominent I descent in hepatic vein	Early in disease e< A on LV inflow Late in disease E > a
	IVC plethora	Pulmonary vein flow = prominent a wave, reduced systolic phase Respiratory variation with decrease of > 25% in Mitral "E" velocity on inspiration	Constant IVRT Absence of significant respiratory variation
Other diagnostic tests	Therapeutic/diagnostic pericardiocentesis	CT or MRI for pericardial thickening	Endomyocardial biopsy

E = early rapid filling wave (peak mitral flow), A = peak velocity of the late filling wave due to atrial contraction

Differential Diagnoses

Aortic Cusp Separation		Aortic Root Diameter	
Normal: 1.5–2.6 cm		**Normal:** 2.0–3.7 cm	
Reduced: Aortic stenosis and subvalvular aortic stenosis, restricted function of left ventricle, hypertrophic obstructive cardiomyopathy, bicuspid valve with secondary calcification		**Enlarged:** Aortic dissection, poststenotic aortic dilatation with aortic stenosis, aortic aneurysm, aneurysm of Sinus of Valsalva, aortic regurgitation	

Right Atrium	Left Atrium	Right Ventricle: Enddiastolic and Endsystolic Diameter
Normal: 2.8–4.0 cm	**Normal:** 2.0–4.0 cm	**Normal:** enddiast.: 0.9–2.6 cm; endsyst.: 1.5–2.2 cm
Enlarged: Tricuspidal valve disease, atrial shunt, pulmonary hypertension, dilated cardiomyopathy, dilated form of coronary heart disease	**Enlarged:** Mitral valve disease, atrial fibrillation, CHD with papillary muscle dysfunction, mitral valve prolapse, mitral valve leaflet rupture, cardiomyopathies, hypertensive heart disease	**Enlarged:** Acute and chronic cor pulmonale, tricuspid regurgitation, pulmonary valve disease, dilated cardiomyopathy, dilated form of coronary heart disease, atrial or ventricular shunt

Left Ventricle: Enddiast. and Endsyst. Diameter	Left Ventricle: Posterior Wall	Left Ventricle: Interventricular Septum
Normal: enddiast.: 3.7–5.6 cm; endsyst.: 2.0–4.0 cm	**Normal:** 0.6–1.1 cm	**Normal:** 0.6–1.1 cm
Enlarged: Dilated cardiomyopathy, dilated form of CHD, posterior wall or septal aneurysm, aortic regurgitation, mitral regurgitation, decompensated hypertensive heart disease	**Enlarged:** Chronic pressure and volume stress, nonobstructive hypertrophic cardiomyopathy, restrictive cardiomyopathies, tumor infiltration **Reduced:** Posterior myocardial infarction, dilated cardiomyopathy	**Enlarged:** Septal hypertrophy in hypertensive heart disease, hypertrophic cardiomyopathies, chronic pressure stress of RV, restrictive cardiomyopathy, tumor infiltration **Reduced:** Septal infarction

EPSS (E Point Septal Separation)	D/E Excursion	E/F-Slope
Normal: 0.2–1.2 cm	**Normal:** 1.8–2.8 cm	**Normal:** 70–150 mm/sec
Enlarged: Restricted function of left ventricle, dilated cardiomyopathy, septal infarction, aortic regurgitation	**Enlarged:** MR/-leaflet rupture, mitral valve prolapse **Reduced:** Mitral stenosis, restricted function of LV, AR	**Reduced:** Mitral stenosis, hypertensive heart disease, myxoma of LA

Abnormal LV Filling Patterns

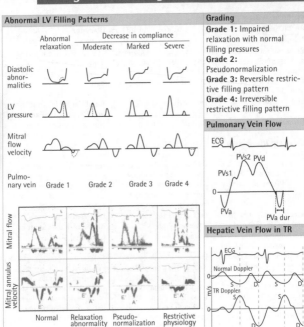

	Abnormal relaxation	Decrease in compliance		
		Moderate	Marked	Severe
Diastolic abnormalities				
LV pressure				
Mitral flow velocity				
Pulmonary vein	Grade 1	Grade 2	Grade 3	Grade 4

	Normal	Relaxation abnormality	Pseudo-normalization	Restrictive physiology
Mitral flow	E A	E A	E A	E A
Mitral annulus velocity	E' A'	E' A'	E' A'	E' A'

Grading

Grade 1: Impaired relaxation with normal filling pressures
Grade 2: Pseudonormalization
Grade 3: Reversible restrictive filling pattern
Grade 4: Irreversible restrictive filling pattern

Pulmonary Vein Flow

ECG

PVs1 PVs2 PVd

0

PVa   PVa dur

Hepatic Vein Flow in TR

ECG

Normal Doppler

0   S   D   S   D

m/s   TR Doppler

0   S   S

D   D

Evaluation of Right Atrial Pressure

IVC	Respiration or "Sniff"	Estimated RA Pressure (mm Hg)
Small (< 1.5 cm)	Collapse	0–5
Normal (1.5–2.5 cm)	↓ > 50%	5–10
Normal	↓ < 50%	11–15
Dilated (> 2.5 cm)	↓ < 50%	16–20
Dilated (with dilated hepatic veins)	No change	>20

Normal Diastolic Indices

E/A ratio	1.32 ± 0.42
Decel. slope	5.0 ± 1.4 m/s^2
IVRT	63 ± 11 ms
Decel. time	150–200 ms
Tau	33 ± 6 ms
E_m	10.3 ± 2.0 cm/s
A_m	5.8 ± 1.6 cm/s
E_m/A_m	2.1 ± 0.9

Classification of Diastolic Dysfunction

	Normal	Mild	Mild to Moderate	Moderate	Severe
Pathophysiology		↓ Relaxation	↓ Relaxation ↑ LVEDP	↓ Relaxation ↓ Compliance ↑ LVEDP	↓ Relaxation ↓↓ Compliance ↑↑ LVEDP
E/A ratio	1–2	< 1	< 1	1–2	> 2.0
E_m/A_m ratio	1–2	< 1	< 1	< 1	> 1
IVRT (ms)	50–100	> 100	N	↓	↓
DT (ms)	150–200	> 200	> 200	150–200	< 150
PV_S/PV_D	≥ 1	$PV_S > PV_D$	$PV_S > PV_D$	$PV_S < PV_D$	$PV_S \ll PV_D$
PV_a (m/s)	< 0.35	< 0.35	≥ 0.35	≥ 0.35	≥ 0.35
a_{dur}–A_{dur} (ms)	< 20	< 20	≥ 20	≥ 20	≥ 20

Parasternal short-axis (PSAx, base)

PSAx (mid-LV)

Apical 4-chamber (A4C)

Apical 2-chamber (A2C)

Apical long-axis (Parasternal long-axis, PLAx)

LAD
RCA
Cx

2.7   Ankle–Brachial Index

Definition	• The Ankle-Brachial Index (ABI) is the ratio of the blood pressure in the lower legs to the blood pressure in the arms. • The ABI is calculated by dividing the higher systolic blood pressure in either the dorsalis pedis or posterior tibial arteries by the higher of the two systolic blood pressures in the arms using the brachial artery.
Step 1	Measure the brachial systolic pressure in both arms
Step 2	Measure the posterior tibial and dorsalis pedis systolic pressures in both legs
Step 3	To calculate the ABI, divide each ankle systolic pressure by the brachial systolic pressure

Classification of Severity of Peripheral Arteries Disease (PAD) Based on ABI	
Normal	ABI > 0.90
Mild	ABI < 0.89 to > 0.60
Moderate	ABI < 0.59 to > 0.40
Severe	ABI < 0.39

Exercise ABI	• Exercise ABI is extremely helpful in making the diagnosis in unclear cases where the ABI at rest is borderline normal or mildly reduced and in situations when the patient presents with exertional lower extremity discomfort from spinal stenosis i.e. pseudoclaudication. • Exercise ABI also may serve as a useful index of disease severity, to assess response to an intervention, and to serially follow up patients. • With exercise challenge (constant speed, constant grade treadmill testing at 2 miles per hour and 12% incline to a maximum of 5 minutes or active pedal plantar flexion), the arterial limb pressure decreases in patients with PAD. A decrease of least 15 mm Hg is considered positive. • The response to exercise in a patient with no PAD is a slight increase or no change in the ankle systolic pressures compared with resting pressures.
Limitations	• ABI may be unreliable in patients with arterial calcification which results in incompressible arteries, because the stiff arteries produce falsely elevated ankle pressure, giving falsely high ABI. • This often is found in patients with diabetes mellitus. ABI values > 1.3 should be considered abnormal and further testing should be done.

2.8 Duplex Sonography

2.8.1 Duplex Sonography: Carotid

Definition	
	• Duplex sonography, a combination of Doppler sonography and B-mode imaging generated by a single transducer, is the diagnostic tool of choice for the initial assessment of carotid disease.
	• This widely available technique allows morphological and functional assessment of the carotid lesion.
	• When performed by trained sonographers using a standard protocol and with ongoing quality assurance, this method provides 90% sensitivity and specificity compared with angiography for detection of severe carotid stenosis.
	• Percent stenosis is determined by systolic and diastolic velocities, with peak end-diastolic velocity > 135 cm/sec and peak end-systolic velocity > 240 cm/sec suggestive of stenosis > 80%.
	• To determine the degree of stenosis present, a complete Doppler evaluation of the artery is necessary.
	• The highest velocity, i.e. peak systolic velocity obtained from a stenosis, is used to classify the degree of narrowing.

Diameter Reduction	Peak Systolic Velocity	End Diastolic Velocity
< 50 %	< 125 cm/s	
50–79 %	≥ 125 cm/s	
80–99 %	≥ 240 cm/s	≥ 135 cm/s
Occlusion	No signal	No signal

Limitation	
	• Duplex carotid scans may yield inadequate images in the following conditions: carotid arteries that bifurcate high, long (> 3 cm) internal carotid artery (ICA) plaques, calcific shadows, and near complete occlusions are reasons for inadequate duplex scans.
	• In these cases, magnetic resonance imaging is of value in differentiating between the two conditions.

2.8.2   Duplex Sonography: Peripheral Arteries

Definition	
	• Native vessel arterial duplex sonography is widely performed.
	• Duplex sonography provides both anatomic and functional information about the arterial system and has been shown to be a reliable technique with fairly good sensitivity and specificity.
	• This examination is generally accepted as a precise method of defining arterial stenoses or occlusions.
	• The sensitivity of duplex sonography to detect occlusions and stenoses in the peripheral arteries has been reported to be 95% and 92%, with specificities of 99% and 97%, respectively.
	• Using a 5.0-7.5 MHz transducer, imaging of the supra- and infrainguinal arteries is performed.
	• The vessels are studied in the sagittal plane, and Doppler velocities are obtained using a 60° Doppler angle

Classification	Percent stenosis
1	Normal
2	1-19 %
3	20-49 %
4	50-99 %
5	Occlusion

• The categories are determined by alterations in the Doppler waveform, as well as ↑ peak systolic velocities. For a stenosis to be classified as 50–99%, for example, the peak systolic velocity must increase by 100% in comparison to the normal segment of artery proximal to the stenosis.

• Arterial duplex sonography (DU) has been used to guide the intervention physician towards appropriate access to a lesion potentially amenable to endovascular therapy, and after endovascular intervention as a means of follow-up.

• Duplex sonography following intervention may overestimate residual stenosis, and may represent a limitation of this technique following intervention.

• Duplex sonography is very helpful in identifying areas of vascular trauma, specifically iatrogenic (pseudoaneurysms occur in up to 7.5% of femoral artery catheterizations and can result in significant complications, including distal embolization into the native arterial system, expansion, extrinsic compression on neurovascular structures, rupture, and hemorrhage).

• Duplex sonography can rapidly and accurately identify these lesions.

• In addition, the use of direct sonography-guided compression or, more recently, sonography-guided thrombin injection can repair these lesions without the need for more invasive surgical procedures.

Limitations	
	• Requires a dedicated vascular sonography laboratory
	• More accurate for above the knee evaluation because tibial arteries are harder to image

2.8.3	Duplex Ultrasonography: Venous
Definition	• Considered to be the best non-invasive diagnostic method for deep vein thrombosis (DVT)
	• Has been evaluated against venography in many studies, showing an average sensitivity and specificity of 97% for proximal deep vein thrombosis.
	• Sensitivity is lower for DVT below the knee, and has been reported to be as low as 75% for calf-vein thrombosis.
	• Duplex sonographic scanning has more recently been used to evaluate the extent of chronic venous insufficiency (CVI).
	• For the diagnosis of DVT, the presence of thrombus on B-mode imaging or compressibility of the vein by the sonography probe has been used.
	• The presence or absence of collateral vessels and partial vessel recanalization can help determine the age of the thrombus.
	• In addition to these data, duplex sonography can provide substantial information in patients with CVI.
	• Compression maneuvers and examination of flow patterns with augmentation can allow systematic evaluation of the saphenofemoral junction and deep, superficial, and perforating veins.
	• Color-flow duplex indicates directionality of blood flow.
	• Venous reflux is then identified by having the patient perform a valsalva maneuver while in 15° reverse Trendelenburg position, or by using rapidly deflating pneumatic cuffs below the level being evaluated to elicit reflux.
	• Incompetent perforator veins are identified and their size measured by holding the transducer directly over the vein while squeezing and releasing the leg.
	• Bidirectionality of flow with compression and release indicates an incompetent perforating vein along with large perforator size.

Three Sonography Techniques are Used Clinically	
Compression sonography	The simplest sonographic criterion for diagnosing venous thrombosis is non-compressibility of the vascular lumen under gentle probe pressure (compression sonography). If no residual lumen is observed, the vein is considered to be fully compressible, which indicates the absence of venous thrombosis.

Duplex ultra-sonography	• Patients are examined in an identical way to that with conventional compression sonography. • In addition, blood flow characteristics are evaluated by using the pulsed Doppler signal. • Blood flow in normal veins is spontaneous and phasic with respiration and can be augmented by manual compression distal to the ultrasound transducer. • When the phasic pattern is absent, flow is defined as continuous, and is suggestive of venous outflow obstruction.
Color flow duplex imaging	• The technique of color-coded Doppler sonography (color Doppler) is identical to duplex sonography. • In color flow sonography, pulsed Doppler signals are used to produce the images. • When a Doppler shift is recognized, it is assigned a color (red or blue) according to its direction, either towards or away from the probe, respectively. • Therefore color Doppler results in a display of flowing blood as a color overlay to the grey-scale sonography image, which makes it easier to identify the veins.
Limitations	• The need for an experienced vascular technologist to perform the examination • Interoperator variability • The inability to accurately visualize the venous system above the inguinal ligament.

2.9   Tilt Table Testing

Definition	• Typically used to diagnose dysautonomia or neurocardiogenic syncope • Patients with symptoms of dizziness or lightheadedness, with or without a loss of consciousness, suspected to be associated with a drop in blood pressure or positional tachycardia, are usual candidates for this test.
Indications	• Unexplained single episode of syncope in a high-risk setting, and recurrent syncope in the absence of heart disease or after cardiac causes have been excluded. • Investigation of recurrent pre-syncope, dizziness or unexplained falls • Patients who have had a single episode of syncope without injury or whose symptoms are obviously vasovagal and diagnosis would not alter treatment.

Criteria for positive test	The test should be considered positive only if the patient's typical symptoms are reproduced and the symptoms are associated with one of three hemodynamic disturbances: • Mixed vasovagal syncope (Type I), in which an abrupt drop in blood pressure is followed by a reduction in heart rate • Cardioinhibitory vasovagal syncope, which describes significant bradycardia (i.e., less than 40 beats per minute for more than 10 seconds or asystole greater than 3 seconds) that either follows (Type IIA) or occurs simultaneously (Type IIB) with a decrease in blood pressure • Vasodepressor syncope (Type III), which manifests with hypotension and without bradycardia
Contraindications	• Unstable cardiovascular disease • Pregnancy • Patient refusal

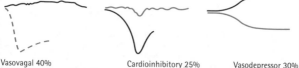

Vasovagal 40%   Cardioinhibitory 25%   Vasodepressor 30%
Red: blood pressure, Black: Heart rate

2.10 Single Photon Emission Computed Tomography

Definition	• Single photon emission computed tomography (SPECT) is a nuclear medicine tomographic imaging technique using gamma rays. • The technique requires injection of a gamma-emitting radioisotope called radionuclide into the bloodstream of the patient. • Because SPECT permits accurate localization in three-dimensional (3D) space, it can be used to provide information about cardiac perfusion. • SPECT imaging performed after stress reveals the distribution of the radiopharmaceutical, and therefore, the relative blood flow to the different regions of the myocardium. • Diagnosis is made by comparing stress images to a further set of images obtained at rest. • ^{201}Thallium, ^{99m}Tc-sestamibi, and ^{99m}Tc-tetrofosmin are 3 routinely used myocardial perfusion imaging tracers for SPECT imaging.

Indications	• Diagnosing the presence, location (coronary territory), and severity of coronary artery disease • Assessing the impact of coronary stenosis on regional perfusion • Distinguishing viable ischemic myocardium from scar tissue • Postmyocardial infarction risk assessment and stratification • Preoperative risk assessment and stratification for major surgery in patients who may be at risk for coronary events • Monitoring effects of treatment after coronary revascularization, medical therapy for congestive heart failure or angina, or lifestyle modification
Limitations	• Perfusion tracers may underestimate severity of CAD • Attenuation artifacts are common • GI tracer interference may be problematic
Clinical utility	• SPECT particularly with ECG-gating is a simple way of assessing myocardial perfusion and left ventricular function within a single study. • The functional parameters are objective, reproducible, and extensively validated. • The continued and substantial growth of SPECT procedures in recent years reflects its clinical utility. • However, proper patient selection, adequate quality control, identification of the technical limitations, and application in appropriate clinical situations are important prerequisites for the optimal utilization of this technique.

Cardiac Views

Short Axis   Apical   Midventricular   Basal

Long Axis   Horizontal   Vertical

2.11   Cardiac CT Angiography

Definition	• Recent advances in computed tomography imaging technology, including the introduction of multidetector row systems, have made imaging of the heart and the coronary arteries feasible.
	• Cardiac CT angiography (CTA) can provide information about coronary anatomy and left ventricular function that can be used in the evaluation of patients with suspected or known coronary artery disease.
	• The ability of a test such as coronary CT angiography to provide incremental diagnostic information that alters management (as contrasted with increasing diagnostic certainty alone) is heavily dependent on the pre-test probability and on the alternative diagnostic strategies considered.
	• The published literature reflects careful selection of study subjects, typically with exclusion of patients who would be expected to have lower quality studies, such as those with irregular heart rates (e.g., atrial fibrillation), obesity, or inability to comply with instructions for breath holding.
	• In these studies, overall sensitivity and specificity on a per patient basis are high and the number of indeterminate studies due to inability to image important coronary segments in the select cohorts represented is < 5%.
	• In most circumstances, a negative coronary CT angiogram rules out significant obstructive coronary disease with a very high degree of confidence, based on the post-test probabilities obtained in cohorts with a wide range of pre-test probabilities.
Indications	• Evaluation of chest pain in an individual with a very low, low, or intermediate pre-test probability of coronary artery disease (CAD) when the individual cannot perform, or has a contraindication to, exercise and chemical stress testing (i.e. exercise treadmill stress test, stress echo, and nuclear stress test [i.e., myocardial perfusion imaging])
	• Exclusion of CAD in an individual with a low or very low pre-test probability of CAD when recent stress test results (i.e., exercise treadmill, stress echo, or nuclear stress test [i.e., myocardial perfusion imaging]) are uninterpretable or equivocal, or when there is a suspicion that the results are falsely positive
	• Exclusion of CAD in an individual with an intermediate pretest probability of CAD when recent stress test results (i.e., exercise treadmill, stress echo, or nuclear stress test [i.e., myocardial perfusion imaging]) are uninterpretable or equivocal, AND when CTA will be performed in lieu of angiography.

Indications	• Exclusion of CAD in a symptomatic individual (e.g., acute chest pain in an emergency department setting), the individual has an intermediate pre-test probability of CAD, there are no changes noted on the ECG, and serial enzymes are negative
	• Evaluation of suspected or known coronary artery anomalies associated with congenital conditions
	• Morphologic evaluation of the coronary arteries in an individual with dilated cardiomyopathy or new onset heart failure, when ischemia is the suspected etiology, and cardiac catheterization and/or nuclear stress test (i.e., myocardial perfusion imaging) have not been performed
	• Pre-operative assessment of coronary arteries in an individual undergoing repair of aortic dissection, aortic aneurysm repair, or valvular surgery AND CTA will be performed in lieu of angiography
	• Post-coronary artery bypass grafting (CABG) when BOTH of the following criteria are met:
	  - Repeat intervention is being considered
	  - Recent coronary angiography has been completed but additional information is needed before a treatment decision can be made

Limitations and safety issues	• The amount of radiation absorbed by the body tissues: median effective radiation dose (for coronary CT angiography with current technology) is approximately 12 mSv. • A number of strategies are being evaluated to lower the radiation dose of coronary CT angiography without affecting diagnostic performance. • The exposure to iodinated contrast agents has the potential to produce allergic reactions and acute renal injury.
Clinical Utility	• CTA is useful in the evaluation of chest pain in an individual with a low or intermediate pre-test probability of CAD. • CTA may be particularly suited for pre-operative assessment of coronary arteries in an individual undergoing repair of aortic dissection, aortic aneurysm repair, or valvular surgery. • However, proper patient selection, adequate quality control, identification of the technical limitations, and application in appropriate clinical situations are important prerequisites for the optimal utilization of this technique.

CT Angiography: Examples

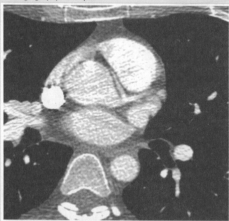

CTA showing coronary arteries

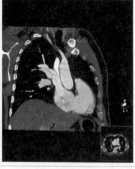

Coronal oblique view showing right upper lobe with anomalous pulmonary venous connection to SVC

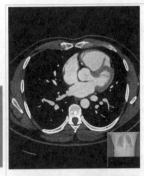

Atrial septal defect on axial view

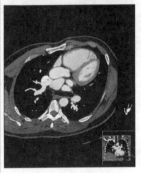

Axial oblique view showing anomalous
pulmonary venous connection

2.12 Cardiac Magnetic Resonance Imaging

Definition	• Cardiac magnetic resonance (CMR) is an imaging technology for the non-invasive assessment of the function and structure of the cardiovasc. system. • Use of ECG-gating and rapid imaging techniques or sequences allows assessment of key functional and morphological features of the cardiovascular system, and this technique has a wide range of clinical applications. • Many of these applications are employed in clinical practice, for example, in the evaluation of congenital heart disease, cardiac masses, the pericardium, right ventricular dysplasia, and hibernating myocardium. • Myocardial perfusion and of valvular and ventricular function are very accurately evaluated with MRI, but competing modalities such as single-photon emission computed tomography (SPECT) imaging and echocardiography are more commonly employed in clinical practice. • Coronary artery imaging is currently more accurately evaluated with other modalities. • One of the main advantages of CMR is the lack of ionizing radiation, which is substantial with SPECT and computed tomography (CT).
Indications	• Assessment of LV and RV size and morphology, systolic and diastolic function, and for characterizing myocardial tissue for the purpose of understanding the etiology of LV systolic or diastolic dysfunction • Patients suspected of amyloidosis or other infiltrative diseases, arrhythmogenic right ventricular dysplasia, or hypertrophic cardiomyopathy • For assessing individuals with valvular heart disease in which evaluation of valvular stenosis, regurgitation, para- or perivalvular masses, perivalvular complications of infectious processes, or prosthetic valve disease is needed. CMR may be useful in identifying serial changes in LV volume or mass in patients with valvular dysfunction • For clin. evaluation of cardiac masses, extracardiac structures, and involvement /characterization of masses in the different. of tumors from thrombi • A noninvasive imaging modality to diagnose patients with suspected pericardial disease. CMR can provide a comprehensive structural and functional assessment of the pericardium and evaluate the physiological consequences of pericardial constriction. • For assessing cardiac structure and function, blood flow, and cardiac and extracardiac conduits in individuals with simple and complex congenital heart disease. Specifically, CMR can be used to identify and characterize congenital heart disease, to assess the magnitude or quantify the severity of intracardiac shunts or extracardiac conduit blood flow, to evaluate the aorta, and to assess the pathologic and physiologic consequences of congenital heart disease on left and right atrial and ventricular function and anatomy.

Contraindications	Patients who have implanted medical devices (e.g. pacemakers or defibrillators, cochlear implants, cerebral aneurysm clips), or who may have iron fragments in their eyes, are not suitable for MRI investigation (orthopaedic pins, mediastinal clips, coronary stents, and the majority of artificial heart valves are safe for scanning)
Special issue	• Use of gadolinium-based contrast agents (GBCAs) has been associated with nephrogenic systemic fibrosis (NSF), a rare, but serious, condition associated in certain patients with kidney dysfunction. • Patients at greatest risk for developing NSF after receiving GBCAs are those with impaired elimination of the drug, including patients with acute kidney injury (AKI) or chronic, severe kidney disease (with a glomerular filtration rate (GFR) < 30 mL/min/1.73m^2). • Higher than recommended doses or repeat doses of GBCAs also appear to increase the risk for NSF.

Current recommendations for use of gadolinium-based contrast agents include	• Do not use three of the GBCA drugs (Magnevist, Omniscan, and Optimark) in patients with AKI or chronic, severe kidney disease. These three GBCA drugs are contraindicated in these patients.
	• Screen patients prior to administration of a GBCA to identify those with AKI or chronic, severe, kidney disease. These patients appear to be at highest risk for NSF.
	• Use the clinical history to screen patients for features of AKI or risk factors for chronically reduced kidney function.
	  - Features of AKI consist of rapid (over hours to days) and usually reversible decrease in kidney function, commonly in the setting of surgery, severe infection, injury, or drug-induced kidney toxicity. Serum creatinine levels and estimated GFR may not reliably assess kidney function in the setting of AKI.
	  - For patients at risk for chronically-reduced kidney function (such as patients over age 60 years, patients with high blood pressure, or patients with diabetes), estimate the kidney function (GFR) with laboratory results.
	• Avoid use of GBCAs in patients suspected or known to have impaired drug elimination unless the need for the diagnostic information is essential and not available with non-contrasted MRI or other alternative imaging modalities.
	• Monitor for signs and symptoms of NSF after a GBCA is administered to a patient suspected or known to have impaired elimination of the drug.
	• Do not repeat administration of any GBCA during a single imaging session.

Cardiac MRI Examples

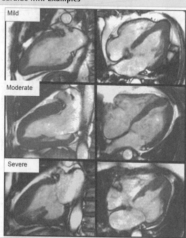

Mild

Moderate

Severe

Examples of mild, moderate, and severe apical HCM. All three patients exhibit the typical asymmetrical apical hypertrophy but this is more subtle in mild HCM and an accurate slice is required to show the apical morphology

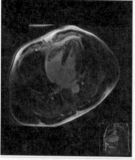

4-chamber delayed enhancement showing apical infarct

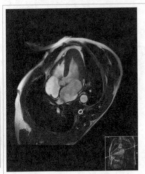

Apical HCM: 4-chamber SSFP image

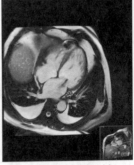

Non-compaction with left atrial enlargement and spin dephasing indicating mitral regurgitation

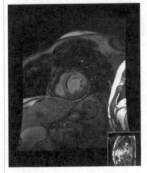

Non viable-myocardium with anteroseptal transmural enhancement indicating irreversible injury and microvascular obstruction

2.13   Cardiac Catheterization

Coronary and Ventricular Anatomy

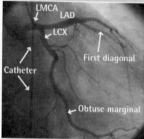

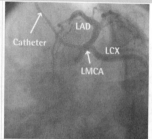

- The fluoroscopy camera (FC) is in the RAO and caudal orientation.
- View is best for showing the anatomy of the proximal LAD and LCX.

- The FC is in the LAO and caudal orientation.
- View is also called the spider view and is best for showing the anatomy of the LMCA and the bifurcation of the LAD and LCX.

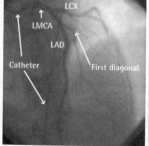

- Camera is in the AP and cranial orientation.
- This view shows the LAD and its branches.

- Camera is in the AP and cranial orientation.
- This view shows the RCA and its branches.

AP = anteroposterior; LAD = left anterior descending; LAO = left anterior oblique; LCX = left circumflex artery; LMCA = left main coronary artery; PDA = posterior descending artery; PLV = posterior left ventricular branch; RAO = right anterior oblique; RCA = right coronary artery.

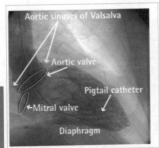

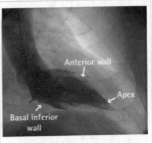

RAO ventriculogram during diastole.   During systole, normal LV function and no MR

Class I Indications for Coronary Angiography	
Asymptomatic or stable angina	• Canadian Cardiovascular Society (CCS) class III and IV on medical therapy • High-risk criteria on noninvasive testing
Acute coronary syndrome	• ST or non-ST elevation MI, high-risk unstable angina, postrevascularization ischemia, successfully resuscitated from sudden cardiac death
Cardiomyopathy	• Evaluation in a patient at risk for CAD
Valvular heart disease	• Before valve surgery in patients at risk for CAD • Assessment of severity of valve disease when noninv. tests are inconclusive • When symptoms or pulmonary artery pressure are out of proportion to severity of mitral regurgitation as assessed by noninvasive testing
Before noncardiac surgery	• Angina unresponsive to adequate medical therapy • UA, particularly before intermediate- or high-risk noncardiac surgery • Acute Myocardial Infarction
Congenital heart disease	• Before surgical correction of congenital heart disease in pat. at risk for CAD • Suspected congenital coronary artery anomalies • Before surgical correction of congenital heart conditions frequently associated with coronary artery anomalies • Unexplained cardiac arrest in a young patient
Other uses	• Diseases affecting the aorta when knowledge of the presence/extent of coronary art. involvement is necessary for management (eg, aortic dissect.) • Hypertrophic CM with angina or when heart surgery is planned

CM = cardiomyopathy, MI = myocardial infarction.
Reprinted from the Journal of the American College of Cardiology, 33, Scanlon, PJ, et al. , ACC/AHA guidelines for coronary angiography, 1756-1824, Copyright 1999, with permission from the American College of Cardiology and the American Heart Association, Inc. Published by Elsevier Science Inc.

Pre-procedure Assessment	
History	• Review symptoms and the indication for the cardiac catheterization.
	• Review the medical history, particularly the history of diabetes, renal disease, lung disease, peripheral arterial disease; previous catheterizations (with type and location of stents); history of CABG and location of grafts; other previous surgeries, particularly femoral/iliac arterial revascularization procedures; history of aortic dissection/aneurysm and aortic surgical procedures
	• History of allergies to i.v. dyes, sedatives, antiplatelet, and anticoag. agents
	• Medication: Is the pat. on antiplatelet, anticoagulant or antidiab. agents?
	• Socioeconomic status, affordability of medications, especially clopidogrel; any expected surgical procedures may influence the choice of bare-metal versus drug-eluting stent.
Physical examination	Vital signs; lung, cardiovascular, abdominal, extremity, and peripheral vascular examination; listen for murmurs and bruits; look for sternotomy, abdominal, and groin scars; examine for distal pulses.
Laboratory and other tests	Complete blood count, coagulation profile, blood chemistry test, and ECG should be obtained; chest radiography, stress-testing results, previous coronary angiograms should be reviewed, if available; review the CT scan in patients with aortic dissection or aneurysms.
Consent	Fully explain the risks and benefits to the patient, including statements about possible complications (see complications table); obtain written informed consent and answer questions asked by the patient or family.

Patients at Increased Risk for Complications after Coronary Angiography		
Increased General Medical Risk	Increased Cardiac Risk	Increased Vascular Risk
• Age older than 70 years • Complex congenital heart disease • Morbid obesity • Cachexia or generalized debilitation • Uncontrolled diabetes • Arterial oxygen desaturation • Severe chronic obstructive lung disease • Renal insufficiency (creatinine > 1.5 mg/dL)	• Three-vessel CAD • Left Main CAD • Functional class IV • Signific. mitral or aortic valve disease or mech. prosthesis • Ejection fraction < 35% • High-risk exercise treadmill testing (hypotension or severe ischemia) • Pulmonary hypertension • Pulmonary artery wedge pressure > 25 mm Hg	• Anticoagulation or bleeding diathesis • Uncontrolled systemic hypertension • Severe peripheral arterial disease • Recent stroke

Relative Contraindications for Diagnostic Cardiac Catheterization

- Acute renal failure
- Chronic renal failure secondary to diabetes
- Active gastrointestinal bleeding
- Unexplained fever, which may be due to infection
- Untreated active infection
- Acute stroke
- Severe anemia
- Severe uncontrolled hypertension
- Severe symptomatic electrolyte imbalance
- Severe lack of cooperation by patient due to psychological or severe systemic illness
- Severe concomitant illness that drastically shortens life expectancy or increases risk of therapeutic interventions
- Refusal of patient to consider definitive therapy such as PTCA, CABG, or valve replacement
- Digitalis intoxication
- Documented anaphylactoid reaction to angiographic contrast media
- Severe peripheral vascular disease limiting vascular access
- Decompensated congestive heart failure or acute pulmonary edema
- Severe coagulopathy
- Aortic valve endocarditis

PTCA = percutaneous transluminal coronary angioplasty; CABG = coronary artery bypass graft; Reprinted from the Journal of the American College of Cardiology, 33, Scanlon, PJ, et al. , ACC/AHA guidelines for coronary angiography, 1756-1824, Copyright 1999, with permission from the American College of Cardiology and the American Heart Association, Inc. Published by Elsevier Science Inc.

Complication Rates for Diagnostic and Therapeutic Catheterization

Event	Diagn. Catheterization (%)[1]	PCI (%)[2,3,4]
Mortality	0.11	0.23
Myocardial infarction	0.05	0.4
Stroke	0.07	–
Arrhythmia	0.38	–
Vascular complications	0.43	3.5
Contrast reaction	0.37	–
Perforation of heart chamber	0.28	–
CABG	–	0.3

PCI = percutaneous coronary intervention

[1] Noto TJ Jr, et al. Cardiac catheterization 1990: A report of the Registry of the Society for Cardiac Angiography and Interventions. Cathet Cardiovasc Diagn. 1991; 24:75-83.

[2] Anderson HV, et al. A contemporary overview of percutaneous coronary interventions. The American College of Cardiology-National Cardiovascular Data Registry (ACC-NCDR). J Am Coll Cardiol, 2002; 39:1096-1103.

[3] Fuchs S, et al. Major bleeding complicating contemporary primary percutaneous interventions-incidence, predictors, and prognostic implications. Cardiovasc Revasc Med. 2009; 10:88-93.

[4] Yang EH, et al. Emergency coronary artery bypass surgery for percutaneous coronary interventions. J Am Coll Cardiol 2005; 46:2004-2009.

Criteria for Performing Combined Right and Left Heart Catheterization	
1. Acute heart failure	5. Myocardial disease
2. Cardiogenic shock	6. Pericardial disease
3. Sudden cardiac death	7. Congenital heart disease
4. Valvular heart disease	8. Pulmonary disease

Pre-treatment for Left Heart Catheterization	
History of contrast allergy	• In current practice, a regimen of prednisone 60 mg the night prior to and 18 mg morning of the procedure (as well as diphenhydramine 50 mg, 1 hour before the procedure) often is used • Low- or iso-osmolar contrast agent should be used
Antiplatelet therapy	• Aspirin 325 mg in all cases undergoing a left heart catheterization • Clopidogrel (300 mg the previous day or 600 mg the day of catheterization) if a revascularization procedure is anticipated • Prasugrel 60 mg or ticagrelor 180 mg can be used instead of clopidogrel for acute coronary syndrom (ACS) patients
Strategies for preventing contrast-induced nephropathy	• Sodium bicarbonate infusion (3 ampules of sodium bicarbonate in 1L of 5% dextrose) at a rate of 3 mL/kg/h for 1 h prior to catheterization and 1 mL/kg/h for 6 h after procedure • Normal saline 1 ml/kg/h i.e 0.9% sodium chloride for 12 h before and after the procedure

Catheters	
Constructed from polyethylene or polyurethane with a fine-wire braid within the wall to allow advancement and directional control (torque) and to prevent kinking. The outer diameter ranges from 4F to 8F, but 5F and 6F catheters are most commonly used for diagnostic angiography.	
Judkins	Right (R) and left (L) catheters
Amplatz	Right (R) and left (L) catheters
Internal Mammary Artery (IMA)	IMA left catheter with an angulated tip that allows engagement of the IMA or an upward takeoff of RCA
Multipurpose	Allow engagement of saphenous vein grafts to the right coronary artery

Classification of Coronary Lesions With Regard to PCI Success

Type A Lesions (high success, > 85%; low risk)

- Discrete (< 10 mm)
- Concentric
- Readily accessible
- Nonangulated segment, < 45°
- Smooth contour
- Little or no calcium
- Less than totally occlusive
- Non-ostial location
- No major side-branch involvement
- Absence of thrombus

Type B Lesions (moderate success, 60%–85%; moderate risk)

- Tubular (10–20 mm length)
- Eccentric
- Moderate tortuosity of proximal segment
- Moderately angulated segment, ≥ 45°, < 90°
- Irregular contour
- Moderate to heavy calcification
- Total occlusion < 3 months old
- Ostial location
- Bifurcation lesion requiring double guidewire
- Some thrombus present

Type C Lesions (low success, < 60%; high risk)

- Diffuse (> 2 cm length)
- Excessive tortuosity of proximal segment
- Extremely angulated segments, ≥ 90°
- Total occlusion > 3 months
- Inability to protect major side branches
- Degenerated vein grafts with friable lesions

Reprinted from the Journal of the American College of Cardiology, 12(2), ACC/AHA Task Force Report, Guidelines for Percutaneous Transluminal Coronary Angioplasty Ryan TJ et al., 529–45, Copyright 1988, with permission from the American College of Cardiology. Published by Elsevier Science Inc.

Thrombolysis in Myocardial Infarction (TIMI) Flow

Contrast Flow	TIMI Grade	Native Vessel Flow	Collateral Flow	Graft Flow
Prompt anterograde flow and rapid clearing	3	3	Excellent	3
Slowed distal filling but full opacification of distal vessel	2	2	Good	2
Small amount of flow but incomplete opacification of distal vessel	1	1	Poor	1
No contrast flow	0	0	No visible flow	0

Reprinted from the Journal of the American College of Cardiology, 33, Scanlon, PJ, et al. , ACC/AHA guidelines for coronary angiography, 1756–1824, Copyright 1999, with permission from the American College of Cardiology and the American Heart Association, Inc. Published by Elsevier Science Inc.

Normal Hemodynamic Values

Chamber	Nl. Press. (mm Hg)	Chamber	Nl. Press. (mm Hg)
Right atrium		Left atrium	
A wave	2–7	A wave	4–16
V wave	2–7	V wave	6–21
Mean	1–5	Mean	2–12
Right ventricle		Left ventricle	
Peak-systole	15–30	Peak-systole	90–140
End-diastole	1–7	End-diastole	6–12
Pulmonary artery		Aorta	
Peak-systole	15–30	Peak-systole	90–140
End-diastole	4–12	End-diastole	60–90
Mean	9–19	Mean	70–105
Wedge (mean)	6–12		

Classification of Valvular Regurgitation by Angiography

+	Minimal regurgitant jet seen; clears rapidly from proximal chamber with each beat
++	Moderate opacification of proximal chamber, clearing with subsequent beats
+++	Intense opacification of proximal chamber, becoming equal to that of the distal chamber
++++	Intense opacification of proximal chamber, becoming more dense than that of the distal chamber throughout the entire series of images obtained

Provocative Testing for Coronary Artery Spasm

General information		• Uses either IV or coronary methylergonovine • Test is both sensitive and specific, but the interpretation is subjective • Must withdraw both nitrates and calcium channel antagonists > 48 h before testing • Women are more sensitive than men to methylergonovine • The intracoronary route is preferable in hypertensive patients and affords the opportunity to separately evaluate the left and right coronary circulations • Risk of inducing severe refractory spasm must be carefully considered prior to performing this provocative maneuver
Contra-indications	Absolute	Pregnancy, severe hypertension, severe left ventricular dysfunction, moderate to severe aortic stenosis and high-grade left main coronary stenosis
	Relative	Uncontrolled or unstable angina, uncontrolled ventricular arrhythmia, recent MI, and advanced coronary disease

Hemodynamic Calculations

Shunt fraction equation	PBF/SBF = $(S_aO_2 - M_vO_2) / (P_vO_2 - P_aO_2)$ PBF = pulmonary blood flow; SBF = systemic blood flow; M_vO_2 = mixed venous O_2 Saturation; S_aO_2 = systemic arterial O_2 Saturation; P_vO_2 = pulmonary venous O_2 Saturation; P_aO_2 = pulmonary arterial O_2 Saturation
Flamm equation	$M_vO_2 = [3 \times (SVC\ O_2\ content) + (IVC\ O_2\ content)] / 4$ SVC = superior vena cava; IVC = inferior vena cava
Hakki Formula (estimated aortic valve area)	AV area (cm²) = CO (L/min) / sqrt[mean AV gradient (mm Hg)] CO = cardiac output; AV= aortic valve
Estimation of mitral valve area	MV area (cm²) = [CO (L/min) x 1000] / [37.7 x HR x DFP x sqrt (mean MV gradient (mm Hg))]; DFP = diastolic filling period; HR = heart rate; MV = mitral valve
Fick equation (estimated cardiac output)	CO (L/min) = O_2 consumption (mL/min) / [AV O_2 Diff (vol%) x 10] AV O_2 Diff = (arterial Saturation - pulmonary Saturation) x 1.36 x Hgb (g/dL); AV = arteriovenous; Hgb = hemoglobin concentration

Hemodynamic Patterns

Aortic Stenosis

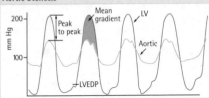

Mitral Stenosis

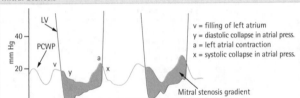

v = filling of left atrium
y = diastolic collapse in atrial press.
a = left atrial contraction
x = systolic collapse in atrial press.

Restrictive Physiology

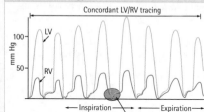

Concordant LV/RV tracing

LV

RV

←——Inspiration——→ ←——Expiration——→

Dip and plateau with equalization of LV and RV pressures

Constrictive Physiology

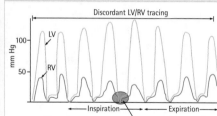

Discordant LV/RV tracing

LV

RV

←——Inspiration——→ ←——Expiration——→

Dip and plateau with equalization of LV and RV pressures

Constrictive Pericarditis vs Restrictive Cardiomyopathy

Parameter	Constrictive Pericarditis	Restrictive Cardiomyopathy
EDP equalization	LVEDP-RVEDP ≤ 5 mm Hg	LVEDP-RVEDP > 5 mm Hg
PA pressure	PASP < 55 mm Hg	PASP > 55 mm Hg
High RVEDP	RVEDP/RVSP > 1/3	RVEDP/RVSP ≤ 1/3
Dip plateau morphology	LV rapid filling wave > 7 mm Hg	LV rapid filling wave ≤ 7 mm Hg
Kussmaul sign	No respiratory variation in mean RA pressure	Normal respiratory variation in mean RA pressure
Respiratory variation of RV/LV pressures	Discordant RV/LV tracing	Concordant RV/LV tracing

RVEDP = right ventricular end-diastolic pressure; LVEDP = left ventricular end-diastolic pressure; PASP = pulmonary artery systolic pressure; RVSP = right ventricular systolic pressure.

3   Cardiovascular Diseases

3.1   Ischemic Heart Disease: Stable Angina Pectoris

3.1.1	Clinical Assessment
History	• Discomfort in the chest, jaw, neck, shoulder, back, or arm • Typically aggravated by exertion or emotional stress • Usually relieved by nitroglycerin • Usually occurs in patients with obstructive coronary artery disease (CAD) but also may occur in patients with severe aortic stenosis, hypertrophic cardiomyopathy, and severe hypertension, even in the absence of CAD.
Physical examination	• Blood pressure, jugular venous pressure • Auscultation (S_4 or S_3 gallop, mitral regurgitant murmur, paradoxically split second heart sound, bibasilar rales or chest wall heave that disappears when the pain subsides are suggestive of coronary artery disease) • Reveals other conditions associated with angina (e.g. valvular heart disease, hypertrophic cardiomyopathy) • Evidence of noncoronary atherosclerotic disease (e.g. carotid bruit, diminished pedal pulse, abdominal aneurysm) increases the likelihood of CAD • Palpation of the chest wall (reveals chest pain caused by musculoskeletal chest wall syndromes)
Initial laboratory tests	Hemoglobin/hematocrit, fasting glucose level, fasting lipid panel, including total cholesterol, HDL-C, triglycerides, and LDL-C
ECG	A normal rest ECG does not exclude severe CAD
Chest radiography	• Reveals pulmonary congestion which may be associated with angina • May also reveal evidence of valvular heart disease, cardiomyopathy, aortic dissection, and/or pericardial effusion

3.1.2 Grading of Angina Pectoris (CCS Classification)

Grade I	• Normal physical activity does not cause angina • Angina with strenuous, rapid, or prolonged exertion at work or recreation.
Grade II	• Slight limitation of normal activity (e.g., walking) • Angina occurs on walking or climbing stairs rapidly, walking uphill, in cold, in wind, under emotional stress, or only during the few hours after awakening • Angina occurs on walking more than 2 blocks on the level and climbing more than one flight of ordinary stairs
Grade III	• Marked limitations of ordinary physical activity • Angina occurs on walking one to two blocks on the level and climbing one flight of stairs in normal conditions and at a normal pace.
Grade IV	• Inability to carry on any physical activity without discomfort • Angina symptoms may be present at rest

3.1.3 Alternative Causes of Chest Pain

Nonischemic cardiovascular	Pulmonary	Gastrointestinal

• Aortic dissection
• Pericarditis
	• Pulmonary embolus
	• Pneumothorax
	• Pneumonia
	• Pleuritis
		• Esophageal
		  - Esophagitis
		  - Spasm
		  - Reflux
		• Biliary
		  - Colic
		  - Cholecystitis
		  - Choledocholithiasis
		• Peptic ulcer
		  - Pancreatitis

Psychiatric	**Chest wall**	
• Anxiety disorders • Hyperventilation • Panic disorder • Primary anxiety • Affective disorders (e.g. depression) • Somatiform disorders • Thought disorders (fixed delusions)	• Costochondritis • Fibrositis • Rib fracture • Sternoclavicular arthritis • Herpes zoster (before the rash)	

Reprinted from the Journal of the American College of Cardiology, 33 (7), Gibbons RJ et al., ACC/ AHA/ACP-ASIM Guidelines for the Management of Patients With Chronic Stable Angina, 2092-2197. Copyright 1999, with permission from the American College of Cardiology and the American Heart Association, Inc. Published by Elsevier Science Inc.

Duke Treadmill Score: Calculation	Interpretation		
Excercise Time (in min on Bruce protocol)	Score	Risk group	Annual mortality
minus (5 x maximum ST-segment deviation (in mm))	≥ 5	Low	0.25 %
minus (4 x angina index, which is: 0 = no angina on test; 1 = angina not limiting; 2 = angina limiting)	-10 to +4	Intermediate	1.25 %
= Total score	≤ -11	High	5.25 %

3.1.4 Noninvasive Risk Stratification

High-Risk (greater than 3% annual mortality rate)	1. Severe resting left ventricular dysfunction (LVEF < 35%) 2. High-risk treadmill score (score ≤ -11) (see above) 3. Severe exercise LV dysfunction (exercise LVEF < 35%) 4. Stress-induced large perfusion defect (particularly if anterior) 5. Stress-induced multiple perfusion defects of moderate size 6. Large, fixed perfusion defect with LV dilation or increased lung uptake (thallium[201]) 7. Stress-induced moderate perfusion defect with LV dilation or increased lung uptake (thallium[201]) 8. Echocardiographic wall motion abnormality (involving > 2 segments) developing at low dose of dobutamine (≤ 10 mg/kg/min) or at a low HR (<120 beats/min) 9. Stress echocardiographic evidence of extensive ischemia
Intermediate-Risk (1%-3% annual mortality rate)	1. Mild-moderate resting LV dysfunction (LVEF = 35% to 49%) 2. Intermediate-risk treadmill score (-11 < score < 5) 3. Stress-induced moderate perfusion defect without LV dilation or increased lung intake (thallium[201]) 4. Limited stress echocardiographic ischemia with a wall motion abnormality, only at higher doses of dobutamine, involving ≤ 2 segments
Low-Risk (less than 1% annual mortality rate)	1. Low-risk treadmill score (score ≥5) 2. Normal or small myocardial perfusion defect at rest or with stress 3. Normal stress echocardiographic wall motion or no change of limited resting wall motion abnormalities during stress

3.1.5   Initial Treatment for Patients with Angina

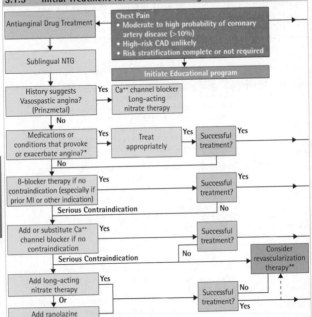

* Conditions that exacerbate or provoke angina

Medications:
* vasodilators
* excessive thyroid replacement
* vasoconstrictors

Other medical problems:
* Profound anemia
* Uncontrolled hypertension
* Hyperthyroidism
* Hypoxemia

Other cardiac problems:
* Tachyarrhythmias
* Bradyarrhythmias
* Valvular heart disease (especially AS)
* Hypertrophic cardiomyopathy

Initial Treatment for Patients with Angina

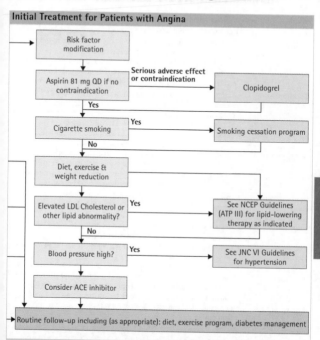

** At any point in this process, based on coronary anatomy, severity of anginal symptoms and patient preferences, it is reasonable to consider evaluation for coronary revascularization. Unless a patient is documented to have left main, three-vessel, or two-vessel coronary artery disease with significant stenosis of the proximal left anterior descending coronary artery, there is no demonstrated survival-advantage associated with revascularization in low-risk patients with chronic stable angina: thus, medical therapy should be attempted in most patients before considering PCI or CABG.

3.1.6   Long-term Therapy for Patients with Angina

Goals	Interventions and Recommendations
Smoking complete cessation	• Smoking cessation and avoidance of exposure to environmental tobacco smoke at work and home is recommended. • Follow-up, referral to special programs, and/or pharmacotherapy (including nicotine replacement) is recommended, as is a stepwise strategy for smoking cessation (Ask, Advise, Assess, Assist, Arrange).
Blood pressure (BP) control goals < 140/90 mm Hg, (< 130/80 mm Hg for patients with diabetes or chronic kidney disease)	• Patients should initiate and/or maintain lifestyle modifications: weight control; increased physical activity; moderation of alcohol consumption; limited sodium intake; and maintenance of a diet high in fresh fruits, vegetables, and low-fat dairy products. • Blood pressure control according to Joint National Conference VII guidelines is recommended (for goals, see left). • For hypertensive patients with well-established coronary artery disease, it is useful to add blood pressure medication as tolerated, treating initially with β-blockers and/or ACE inhibitors, with addition of other drugs as needed to achieve target blood pressure.
Lipid management LDL-C should be < 100 mg/dL, reduction of LDL-C < 70 mg/dL or high-dose statin therapy is reasonable.	• Dietary therapy for all patients should include reduced intake of saturated fats (to less than 7% of total calories), trans-fatty acids, and cholesterol (to less than 200 mg per day). • Adding plant stanol/sterols (2 g per day) and/or viscous fiber (> 10 g per day) is reasonable to further lower LDL-C. • Daily physical activity and weight management are recommended for all patients. • For all patients, encouraging consumption of omega-3 fatty acids in the form of fish* or in capsule form (1 g per day) for risk reduction may be reasonable. For treatment of elevated triglycerides (TG), higher doses are usually necessary for risk reduction. • Recommended lipid management includes assessment of a fasting lipid profile

	If baseline LDL-C is ≥ 100 mg/dL ⇒ LDL-lowering drug therapy should be initiated in addition to therapeutic lifestyle changes. When LDL-lowering medications are used in high-risk or moderately high-risk persons, it is recommended that intensity of therapy be sufficient to achieve a 30% to 40% reduction in LDL-C levels. **Therapeutic options for LDL-C-lowering therapy:** statins or resin**	If on-treatment LDL-C is ≥ 100 mg/dL ⇒ LDL-lowering drug therapy should be intensified.	If baseline LDL-C is 70 to 100 mg/dL ⇒ it is reasonable to treat LDL-C to less than 70 mg per dL
If TG are 200 to 499 mg/dL ⇒ non-HDL-C*** should be < 130 mg/dL. Further reduction of non-HDL-C*** to < 100 mg/dL is reasonable, if TG are ≥ 200-499 mg/dL.	**Therapeutic options to reduce non-HDL-C are:** • Niacin can be useful as a therapeutic option to reduce non-HDL-C (after LDL-C-lowering therapy)# or • Fibrate therapy as a therapeutic option can be useful to reduce non-HDL-C (after LDL-C-lowering therapy). • If TG are ≥ 500 mg/dL, therapeutic options to lower the TG to reduce the risk of pancreatitis are fibrate or niacin; these should be initiated before LDL-C-lowering therapy. • The goal is to achieve non-HDL-C < 130 mg/dL if possible.		
	The following lipid management strategies can be beneficial: • If LDL-C < 70 mg/dL is the chosen target, consider drug titration to achieve this level to minimize side effects and cost. • When LDL-C < 70 mg/dL is not achievable because of high baseline LDL-C-levels, it generally is possible to achieve reductions of > 50% in LDL-C-levels by either statins or LDL-C-lowering drug combinations. • Drug combinations are beneficial for patients on lipid lowering therapy who are unable to achieve LDL-C < 100 mg/dL.		

Physical activity Physical activity of 30 to 60 minutes, 7 days per week (minimum 5 days per week) is recommended.	• All patients should be encouraged to obtain 30 to 60 minutes of moderate-intensity aerobic activity, such as brisk walking, on most, preferably all days of the week, supplemented by an increase in daily activities (such as walking breaks at work, gardening, or household work). • The patient's risk should be assessed with a physical activity history. Where appropriate, an exercise test is useful to guide the exercise prescription (see page 32 and for further information Exercise Testing Guideline) • Medically supervised programs (cardiac rehab.) are recommended for at-risk patients (e.g., recent acute coronary syndrome or revascul., HF). • Expanding physical activity to include resistance training on 2 days per week may be reasonable.
Weight management BMI 18,5-24,9 kg/m² The initial goal of weight loss therapy should be to gradually reduce body weight by approximately 10% from baseline.	• BMI and waist circumference should be assessed regularly. • On each patient visit, it is useful to consistently encourage weight maintenance/reduction through an appropriate balance of physical activity, caloric intake, and formal behavioral programs when indicated. • If waist circumference is ≥ 35 inches (89 cm) in women or ≥ 40 inches (102 cm) in men ⇒ initiate lifestyle changes and consider treatment strategies for metabolic syndrome as indicated. • Some male patients can develop multiple metabolic risk factors when the waist circumference is only marginally increased (e.g., 37- 40 inches [94 to 102 cm]). Such persons may have a strong genetic contribution to insulin resistance. They should benefit from changes in life habits, similarly to men with categorical increases in waist circumference.
Diabetes management HbA₁c < 7 %	• Diabetes management should include lifestyle and pharmacotherapy measures to achieve a near-normal HbA₁c. • Vigorous modification of other risk factors (e.g., physical activity, weight management, blood pressure control, and cholesterol management) as recommended should be initiated and maintained
Antiplatelet agents/ Anticoagulants	• Aspirin should be started at 75-162 mg per day and continued indefinitely in all patients unless contraindicated. • Use of warfarin in conjunction with aspirin and/or clopidogrel is associated with an increased risk of bleeding ⇒ close monitoring.
ACE inhibitors (ACEI), Angiotensin-receptor-blockers, Aldosterone blockers	• ACEI should be started and continued indefinitely in all patients with left ventricular ejection fraction ≤ 40% and in those with hypertension, diabetes, or chronic kidney disease unless contraindicated. • ACEI should be started and continued indefinitely in pat. who are not at lower risk (defined as those with normal left ventricular ejection fraction in whom cardiovascular risk factors are well controlled and revascularization has been performed), unless contraindicated.

ACE inhibitors (ACEI), Angiotensin-receptor-blockers, Aldosterone blockers	• It is reasonable to use ACE inhibitors among lower-risk patients with mildly reduced or normal left ventricular ejection fraction, in whom cardiovascular risk factors are well controlled and revascularization has been performed.
	• Angiotensin-receptor-blockers are recommended for patients who have hypertension; indications for (but are intolerant of) ACE inhibitors; heart failure; or had a myocardial infarction, with left ventricular ejection fraction ≤ 40%.
	• Angiotensin-receptor-blockers may be considered in combination with ACE inhibitors for heart failure due to left ventricular systolic dysfunction.
	• Aldosterone blockade is recommended for use in post-MI patients without significant renal dysfunction## or hyperkalemia who are already receiving therapeutic doses of an ACE inhibitor and a β-blocker, have a left ventricular ejection fraction ≤ 40%, and have either diabetes or heart failure.
β–Blockers	It is beneficial to start and continue β-Blocker therapy indefinitely in all pat. who have had MI, acute coronary syndrome, or left ventricular dysfunction with or without HF symptoms, unless contraindicated.
Influenza vaccination	An annual influenza vaccination is recommended for patients with cardiovascular disease.
Chelation therapy	Chelation therapy (intravenous infusions of ethylenediamine tetraacetic acid (EDTA)) is not recommended for the treatment of chronic angina or arteriosclerotic cardiovascular disease and may be harmful because of its potential to cause hypocalcemia.

ACE = angiotensin-converting enzyme, BP = blood pressure, TG = triglycerides, BMI = body-mass index, HbA$_{1c}$ = major fraction of adult hemoglobin, MI = myocardial infarction, HF = heart failure, RI = renal insufficiency; *Pregnant and lactating women should limit their intake of fish to minimize exposure to methylmercury.** The use of resin is relatively contraindicated when TG > 200 mg/dL; *** Non-HDL-Cholesterol (Non-HDL-C) = Total cholesterol minus HDL cholesterol. #The combination of high-dose statin and fibrate can increase risk for severe myopathy. Statin doses should be kept relatively low with this combination. Dietary supplement niacin must not be used as a substitute for prescription niacin. ## Creatinine should be < 2.5 mg/dL in men and < 2.0 mg/dL in women. Potassium should be < 5.0 mEq/ L

3.2   Acute Coronary Syndrome (ACS)

3.2.1   Definition of ACS

- ACS has evolved as a useful operational term to refer to any constellation of clinical symptoms that are compatible with acute myocardial ischemia.
- The spectrum of acute ischemia-related syndromes ranges from unstable angina to acute myocardial infarction (MI) with (STEMI) or without (NSTEMI) ST-segment elevation.

Comparison: Previous and Current Definitions of the Entities of the ACS

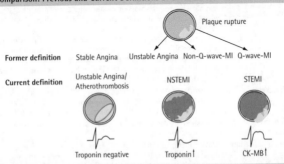

The Clinical Diagnosis Relies on the Combination of at Least Two of the Following:

• History (angina or anginal aquivalent)	• Typical rise or fall of cardiac biomarkers
• Acute ischemic ECG changes	• Absence of another identifiable etiology

3.2.2   Alternative Causes of Chest Pain
See →74

3.2.3   ECG Diagnostics of ACS
See →31

3.2.4   Clinical Suspicion of ACS

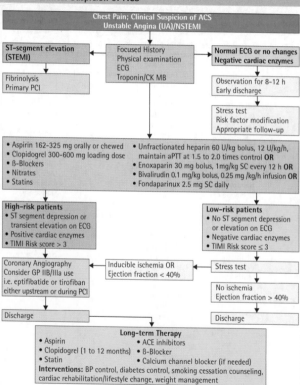

Chest Pain; Clinical Suspicion of ACS
Unstable Angina (UA)/NSTEMI

Focused History
Physical examination
ECG
Troponin/CK MB

ST-segment elevation (STEMI)
- Fibrinolysis
- Primary PCI

Normal ECG or no changes Negative cardiac enzymes
Observation for 8–12 h
Early discharge

Stress test
Risk factor modification
Appropriate follow-up

- Aspirin 162–325 mg orally or chewed
- Clopidogrel 300–600 mg loading dose
- ß-Blockers
- Nitrates
- Statins

- Unfractionated heparin 60 U/kg bolus, 12 U/kg/h, maintain aPTT at 1.5 to 2.0 times control **OR**
- Enoxaparin 30 mg bolus, 1mg/kg SC every 12 h **OR**
- Bivalirudin 0.1 mg/kg bolus, 0.25 mg /kg/h infusion **OR**
- Fondaparinux 2.5 mg SC daily

High-risk patients
- ST segment depression or transient elevation on ECG
- Positive cardiac enzymes
- TIMI Risk score > 3

Low-risk patients
- No ST segment depression or elevation on ECG
- Negative cardiac enzymes
- TIMI Risk score ≤ 3

Coronary Angiography Consider GP IIB/IIIa use i.e. eptifibatide or tirofiban either upstream or during PCI

Inducible ischemia OR Ejection fraction < 40%

Stress test

No ischemia
Ejection fraction > 40%

Discharge

Discharge

Long-term Therapy
- Aspirin
- Clopidogrel (1 to 12 months)
- Statin
- ACE inhibitors
- ß-Blocker
- Calcium channel blocker (if needed)

Interventions: BP control, diabetes control, smoking cessation counseling, cardiac rehabilitation/lifestyle change, weight management

3.2.5	Biochemical Cardiac Markers for the Evaluation and Management of Patients With Suspected ACS				
Marker	Advantages	Disadvantages	PoCT avai- lable	Comment	Clinical recom- mendations
Cardiac troponins	• Powerful tool for risk stratification • Greater sensitivity and specificity than CK-MB • Detection of recent MI up to 2 weeks after onset • Useful for selection of therapy • Detection of reperfusion	• Low sensitivity in very early phase of MI (< 6 h after symptom onset), requires repeat measure- ment at 8 h to 12 h, if negative • Limited ability to detect late minor reinfarc- tion	YES	Data on diagnos- tic performance and potential therapeutic implications increasingly available from clinical trials	Useful as a single test to efficiently diagnose NSTEMI (incl. minor myo- cardial damage), with serial measurements. **Caveat:** Clinicians should familiarize them- selves with dia- gnostic "cutoffs" used in their local hospital laboratory
CK–MB	• Rapid, cost- efficient, accurate assays • Ability to detect early reinfarction	• Loss of speci- ficity in setting of skeletal muscle disease or injury, including surgery • Low sensitivity during very early MI (< 6 h after symptom onset) or later after symptom onset (> 36 h) and for minor myocar- dial damage (detectable with troponins)	YES	Familiar to majority of clinicians	Prior standard and still acceptable diagnostic test in most clinical circumstances

| Myo-globin | • High sensitivity
• Useful in early detection of MI
• Detection of reperfusion
• Most useful in ruling out MI | • Very low specificity in setting of skeletal muscle injury or disease
• Rapid return to normal range limits sensitivity for later presentations | YES | More convenient early marker than CK-MB isoforms because of greater availability of assays for myoglobin; rapid-release kinetics make myoglobin useful for non-invasive monitoring of reperfusion in patients with established MI |

*PoCT= Point of care test; Reprinted from the Journal of the American College of Cardiology, 50 (7), Anderson JL, et al., ACC/AHA 2007 Guidelines for the Management of Patients With Unstable Angina/ Non-ST-Elevation Myocardial Infarction, e1-e157. Copyright 2007, with permission from the American College of Cardiology Foundation and the American Heart Association. Published by Elsevier Inc.

3.2.6   Cardiac Enzyme Kinetics

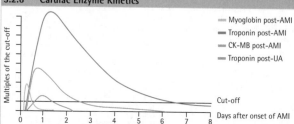

Legend:
- Myoglobin post-AMI
- Troponin post-AMI
- CK-MB post-AMI
- Troponin post-UA

Y-axis: Multiples of the cut-off
X-axis: Days after onset of AMI (0 1 2 3 4 5 6 7 8)
Cut-off line labeled

3.2.7   Differential Diagnosis of High Troponin Level

- Severe heart failure
- Aortic dissection
- Hypertrophic obstructive cardiomyopathy
- Heart contusion, -ablation
- Hypothyroidism
- Defibrillation/Cardioversion
- Tachycardia/Bradycardia
- Hypertensive crisis
- Tako-Tsubo syndrome
- Renal insufficiency
- Stroke
- Severe sepsis
- Rhabdomyolysis
- Respiratory insufficiency
- Intoxication

3.3 Unstable Angina/NSTEMI (Non ST–segment Elevation Myocardial Infarction)

3.3.1 Principal Presentations of Unstable Angina

Rest angina	Angina occurring at rest and prolonged, usually > 20 min
New-onset angina	New-onset angina of at least CCS class III severity
Increasing angina	Previously-diagnosed angina that has become distinctly more frequent, longer in duration, or lower in threshold (i.e., increased by 1 or more CCS class to at least CCS class III severity)

Reprinted from the Journal of the American College of Cardiology, 50 (7), Anderson JL, et al., ACC/AHA 2007 Guidelines for the Management of Patients With Unstable Angina/Non–ST-Elevation Myocardial Infarction, e1-e157. Copyright 2007, with permission from the American College of Cardiology Foundation and the American Heart Association. Published by Elsevier Inc.

3.3.2 UA/NSTEMI: Short-Term Risk of Death or Nonfatal MI*

	High Risk	Intermediate Risk	Low Risk
	At least 1 of the following features (ff) must be present	No high risk feature, but must have 1 of the following features (ff)	No high- or intermed.-risk feature but may have any of the ff
History	Accelerating tempo of ischemic symptoms in preceding 48 h	Prior MI, peripheral or cerebrovascular disease, or CABG; prior aspirin use	
Character of pain	Prolonged ongoing (> 20 min) rest pain	• Prolonged (> 20 min) rest angina, now resolved, with moderate or high likelihood of CAD • Rest angina (≥ 20 min) or relieved with rest or SL NG • Nocturnal angina • New-onset or progressive CCS class III or IV angina in the past 2 weeks without prolonged (> 20 min) rest pain but with intermediate or high likelihood of CAD	• Increased angina frequency, severity, or duration • Angina provoked at a lower threshold • New onset angina, with onset 2 weeks to 2 months prior to presentation
Clinical findings	• Pulmonary edema, most likely due to ischemia • New or worsening MR murmur, S₃ or new/worsening rales • Hypotension, brady-, tachycardia • Age > 75 years	Age greater than 70 years	

ECG	• Angina at rest with transient ST-segment changes greater than 0.5 mm • Bundle-branch block, new or presumed new sustained VT	• T-wave changes • Pathological Q waves or resting ST-depression less than 1 mm in multiple lead groups (anterior, inferior, lateral)	Normal or unchanged ECG
Cardiac markers	Elevated cardiac Tropopin T, Troponin I, or CK-MB (e.g., TnT or TnI greater than 0.1 ng per ml)	Slightly elevated cardiac TnT, or CK-MB (e.g., TnT greater than 0.01 but less than 0.1 ng per ml)	Normal

* Estimation of the short-term risks of death and nonfatal cardiac ischemic events in UA (or NSTEMI) is a complex multivariable problem that cannot be fully specified in a table such as this; therefore, this table is meant to offer general guidance and illustration rather than rigid algorithms; NG = nitroglycerin; SL = sublingual

Reprinted from the Journal of the American College of Cardiology, 50 (7), Anderson JL, et al., ACC/AHA 2007 Guidelines for the Management of Patients With Unstable Angina/Non–ST-Elevation Myocardial Infarction, e1–e157. Copyright 2007, with permission from the American College of Cardiology Foundation and the American Heart Association. Published by Elsevier Inc.

3.3.3   TIMI Score for Patients with UA/NSTEMI

Description of the TIMI Risk Score (Thrombolysis In Myocardial Infarction)

The TIMI Risk Score is determined by the sum of the presence of 7 variables at admission. 1 point is given for each of the follwowing variables:

- 65 y or older
- At least 3 risk factors for CAD
- Prior coronary stenosis of 50% or more
- ST-segment deviation on ECG
- At least 2 anginal events in prior 24h
- Use of aspirin in prior 7 d
- Elevated serum cardiac biomarkers

The TIMI Risk Score for 0-1 points is 4.7%, for 2 points 8.3%, for 3 points 13.2%, for 4 points 19.9%, for 5 points 26.2% and for 6-7 points 40.9%. The percentage values refer to all cause mortality, new or recurrent MI, or severe recurrent ischemia requiring urgent revascularization through 14 d after randomization.

Prior coronary stenosis of 50% or more remained relatively insensitive to missing information and remained a significant predictor of events

3.3.4   Selection of Initial Treatment Strategy

Invasive	Conservative

- Recurrent angina or ischemia at rest or with low-level activities despite intensive medical therapy
- Elevated cardiac biomarkers (Troponin T or I)
- New or presumably-new ST-segment depression
- Signs or symptoms of heart failure or new or worsening mitral regurgitation
- High-risk findings from noninvasive testing
- Hemodynamic instability
- Sustained ventricular tachycardia
- PCI within 6 months
- Prior CABG
- High risk score (e.g., TIMI, GRACE)
- Reduced left ventricular function (LVEF < 40%)

- Low risk score (e.g., TIMI, GRACE)
- Patient or physician preference in the absence of high-risk features

TIMI = Thrombolysis In Myocardial Infarction; GRACE = Global Registry of Acute Coronary Events; PCI = percutaneous coronary intervention;

3.3.5 Recommendations for Anti-Ischemic Therapy: Continuing Ischemia/Other Clinical High-Risk Features Present*

Bed/chair rest	With continuous ECG monitoring
Oxygen	Supplemental with an arterial saturation less than 90%, respiratory distress, or other high-risk features for hypoxemia.
Pulse oximetry	Can be useful for continuous measurement of S_aO_2
Nitroglycerin (NTG)	• 0.4 mg sublingually every 5 min for a total of 3 doses; afterward, assess need for IV NTG • IV for first 48 h after UA/NSTEMI for treatment of persistent ischemia, HF, or hypertension • Decision to administer NTG IV and dose should not preclude therapy with other mortality-reducing interventions such as β-Blockers or ACE inhibitors
β-Blockers	Via oral route within 24 h without a contraindication (e.g., HF) irrespective of concomitant performance of PCI
Non-dihydro-pyridine calcium channel blocker	When β-Blockers are contraindicated e.g., verapamil or diltiazem should be given as initial therapy in the absence of severe LV dysfunction or other contraindications
ACE inhibitor	Via oral route within first 24 h in patients with pulmonary congestion or LVEF ≤ 0.40, in the absence of hypotension (systolic blood pressure < 100 mm Hg or < 30 mm Hg below baseline) or known contra-indications to that class of medications
Angiotensin-receptor blockers (ARB)	Should be administered to UA/NSTEMI patients who are intolerant of ACE inhibitors and have either clinical or radiological signs of heart failure or LVEF ≤ 0.40

* Recurrent angina and/or ischemia-related ECG changes (0.05 mV or greater ST-segment depression or bundle-branch block) at rest or with low-level activity; or ischemia associated with HF symptoms, S_3 gallop, or new or worsening mitral regurgitation; or hemodynamic instability or depressed LV function (LVEF< 0.40 on noninvasive study); or serious ventricular arrhythmia.

ACE = angiotensin-converting enzyme; ARB = angiotensin receptor blocker; HF = heart failure; IV = intravenous; LV = left ventricular; LVEF = left ventricular ejection fraction; NTG = nitroglycerin; MI = myocardial infarction; PCI = percutaneous coronary intervention; UA/NSTEMI = unstable angina/non-ST-elevation myocardial infarction.;

Reprinted from the Journal of the American College of Cardiology, 50 (7), Anderson JL, et al., ACC/AHA 2007 Guidelines for the Management of Patients With Unstable Angina/Non–ST-Elevation Myocardial Infarction, e1–e157. Copyright 2007, with permission from the American College of Cardiology Foundation and the American Heart Association. Published by Elsevier Inc.

3.3.6   Medications Used for Stabilized UA/NSTEMI Patients

Anti-Ischemic and Antithrombotic/ Antiplatelet Agents	Drug Action
Aspirin	Antiplatelet
Clopidogrel	Antiplatelet when aspirin is contraindicated
Clopidogrel	In combination with aspirin for 1-12 months
ACE inhibitors	EF less than 0.40 or heart failure
Nitrates	Antianginal
Calcium channel blockers (short-acting dihydropyridine antagonists should be avoided)	Antianginal
Dipyridamole	Antiplatelet

Agents for Secondary Prevention and Other Indications	Risk Factor
HMG-CoA reductase inhibitors	LDL cholesterol > 70 mg/dL
Fibrates	HDL cholesterol < 40 mg/dL
Niacin	HDL cholesterol < 40 mg/dL
Niacin or fibrate	Triglycerides 200 mg/dL
Antidepressant	Treatment of depression
Treatment of hypertension	Blood pressure > 140/90 mm Hg (or > 130/80 mm Hg if kidney disease or diabetes present)
Treatment of diabetes	HbA$_{1c}$ > 7%
Hormone therapy (initiation)	Postmenopausal state
Hormone therapy (continuation)	Postmenopausal state
COX-2 inhibitor or NSAID	Chronic pain

ACE-I = angiotensin-converting enzyme inhibitor; CHF = congestive heart failure; COX-2 = cyclooxygenase 2; EF = ejection fraction; HDL = high-density lipoprotein; HMG-CoA = hydroxymethylglutaryl-coenzyme A; INR = international normalized ratio; LDL = low-density lipoprotein; NSAID = nonsteroidal anti-inflammatory drug; NSTEMI = non-ST-segment elevation myocardial infarction; UA = unstable angina;

3.4   STEMI
(ST-Segment Elevation Myocardial Infarction)

3.4.1	Clinical Assessment
History	• Chest discomfort with or without radiation to the arms(s), back, neck, jaw, or epigastrium • Shortness of breath, weakness, diaphoresis, nausea, lightheadedness • Women and elderly may present with atypical symptoms such as fatigue, malaise, not feeling well etc.
Physical examination	• Airway, Breathing, Circulation (ABC) • Vital signs, general appearance • Presence or absence of jugular venous distension • Pulmonary auscultation for rales • Cardiac auscultation for murmurs and gallops (S_3, S_4) • Presence or absence of stroke • Presence or absence of pulses • Presence or absence of systemic hypoperfusion
Initial laboratory tests	• Serum biomarkers for cardiac damage (do not wait for results to proceed with re-perfusion strategy) • Complete blood count with platelet count • INR (international normalized ratio) • Activated partial thromboplastin time • Electrolytes and magnesium • Blood urea nitrogen (BUN) • Creatinine • Glucose • Serum lipids

3.4.2   Suspected STEMI

Suspected STEMI

- Obtain ECG within 10 minutes of arrival to ED
- Confirm STEMI by ECG (> 1 mm ST segment elevation in two contiguous leads, new LBBB)
- Brief focused history
- Aspirin 162-325 mg chewed

- Clopidogrel 300 mg loading dose
- ß-Blockers*
- Nitrates for ongoing pain, elevated SBP, HF
- Morphine for pain

Assess
- Time since onset of symptoms
- Risk of fibrinolysis
- Time required for transport to a skilled PCI center

Determine whether fibrinolysis or an invasive strategy is preferred
If presentation is < 3 hours and there is no delay to an invasive strategy, there is no preference for either strategy

Fibrinolysis is generally preferred if:
- Early presentation
  (≤ 3 hours from symptom onset and delay to invasive strategy; see below)
- Invasive strategy is not an option
  - Catheterization laboratory occupied or not available
  - Vascular access difficulties
  - Lack of access to a skilled PCI laboratory
- Delay to invasive strategy
  - Prolonged transport
  - (Door-to-Balloon) – (Door-to-Needle) time is > 1 hour
  - Medical contact-to-balloon or door-to-balloon time is > 90 minutes

Catheteriz. ± PCI is generally preferred if:
- Skilled PCI laboratory available with surgical backup
  - Medical contact-to-balloon or door to-balloon is < 90 minutes
  - (Door-to-Balloon) – (Door-to-Needle) < 1 h
- High-risk from STEMI
  - Cardiogenic shock
  - Killip class is ≥ 3
- Contraindications to fibrinolysis, including increased risk of bleeding and intracranial hemorrhage
- Late presentation
  (The symptom onset was > 3 hours ago)
- Diagnosis of STEMI is in doubt

* Oral ß-Blocker therapy should be initiated in the first 24 hours for patients who do not have any of the following: 1) signs of heart failure, 2) evidence of a low output state, 3) increased risk* for cardiogenic shock, or 4) other relative contraindications to ß-Blockade (PR interval greater than 0.24 seconds, second- or third-degree heart block, active asthma, or reactive airway disease

ED = Emergency department, SBP = systolic blood pressure;
Reprinted from the Journal of the American College of Cardiology , Antman EM et al., ACC/AHA Guidelines for the Management of Patients With ST-Elevation Myocardial Infarction, e1-e211. Copyright 2004, with permission from the American College of Cardiology Foundation and the American Heart Association, Inc. Published by Elsevier Inc.

3.4.3 Dosage of Fibrinolytic Agents

Alteplase	IV bolus 15 mg, infusion 0.75 mg/kg times 30 min (maximum 50 mg), then 0.5 mg/kg; not to exceed 35 mg over the next 60 min to an overall maximum of 100 mg
Reteplase	10 U IV over 2 min; 30 min after the first dose, give 10 U IV over 2 min
Streptokinase	1.5 million U IV over 30-60 min
Tenecteplase	IV bolus over 10-15 seconds, 30 mg for body weight less than 60 kg; 35 mg for 60-69 kg; 40 mg for 70-79 kg; 45 mg for 80-89 kg; 50 mg for 90 kg or more

3.4.4 Contraindications to Fibrinolysis

Absolute Contraindications

- Any prior intracranial hemorrhage
- Known structural cerebrovascular lesion (e.g., arteriovenous malformation)
- Known malignant intracranial neoplasm (primary or metastatic)
- Ischemic stroke within 3 months EXCEPT acute ischemic stroke within 3 hours
- Suspected aortic dissection
- Active bleeding or bleeding diathesis (excluding menses)
- ignificant closed-head or facial trauma within 3 months

Relative Contraindications

- History of chronic, severe, poorly controlled hypertension
- Severe uncontrolled hypertension on presentation (syst. BP > 180 mm Hg or diast. BP > 110 mm Hg)
- History of prior ischemic stroke greater than 3 months, dementia, or known intracranial pathology not covered in contraindications
- Traumatic or prolonged (> 10 minutes) CPR or major surgery (within less than 3 weeks)
- Recent (within 2 to 4 weeks) internal bleeding
- Noncompressible vascular punctures
- For streptokinase/anistreplase: prior exposure (> 5 d ago) or prior allergic reactions to these agents
- Pregnancy
- Active peptic ulcer
- Current use of anticoagulants: the higher the INR, the higher the risk of bleeding

3.4.5 Guidelines for Medical Management of STEMI (ACC/AHA)

Fibrinolysis	Class I	Ischemia symptoms, ST elevation or LBBB < 12 h from symptom onset, age < 75 years
	Class IIa	Same as class I, age ≥ 75 y
	Class IIb	Same as class I and IIA > 12–24 h from symptom onset, BP > 180/110 mm Hg with high risk MI
	Class III	ST elevation, time to therapy > 24 h, symptoms resolved
Aspirin	Class I	Initially 162–325 mg/d; Maintenance 75–162 mg/d indefinitely
Clopidogrel	Class I	75 mg per day orally should be added to aspirin in patients with STEMI regardless of whether they undergo reperfusion with fibrinolytic therapy or do not receive reperfusion therapy

Antithrombotics: Class I - Patients undergoing reperfusion with fibrinolytics should receive anticoagulant therapy for a minimum of 48 hours and preferably for the duration of the index hospitalization, up to 8 days (regimens other than UFH are recommended if anticoagulant therapy is given for more than 48 hours because of the risk of heparin-induced thrombocytopenia with prolonged UFH treatment.

Heparin (unfractionated)	Class I	Patients undergoing primary PCI or bypass surgery. Patients undergoing reperfusion with fibrinolytics should receive anticoagulant therapy for a minimum of 48 h. UFH (initial intravenous bolus 60 U per kg [maximum 4000 U]) followed by an intravenous infusion of 12 U per kg per h (maximum 1000 U per h) initially, adjusted to maintain the activated partial thromboplastin time at 1.5 to 2.0 times control (approximately 50 to 70 s)
	Class IIa	Eight days for patients not receiving reperfusion therapy (regimens other than UFH (preferable)
	Class IIb	Patients undergoing reperfusion therapy with streptokinase
LMWH	Class I	Enoxaparin (provided the serum creatinine is < 2.5 mg/dL in men and 2.0 mg/dL in women); patients < 75 y. For patients less than 75 y of age, an initial 30 mg intravenous bolus is given, followed 15 minutes later by subcutaneous injections of 1.0 mg per kg every 12 h; for patients at least 75 y of age, the initial intravenous bolus is eliminated and the subcutaneous dose is reduced to 0.75 mg per kg every 12 h

Fondaparinux	Class I	Fondaparinux (provided the serum creatinine is < 3.0 mg/dL): initial dose 2.5 mg IV; subsequently SC of 2.5 mg once daily Maintenance dosing with fondaparinux should be continued for the duration of hospitalization, up to 8 days
	Class III	Because of the risk of catheter thrombosis, fondaparinux should not be used as the sole anticoagulant to support PCI
GP-IIb/IIIa-inhibitors	Class IIa	PCI/abciximab
	Class IIb	PCI/eptifibatide, tirofiban
β-Blockers	Class I	Orally in patients without contraindications
	Class IIa	IV in patients without contraindications
	Class III	IV β-Blockers should not be administered with: • signs of heart failure • evidence of a low output state • increased risk for cardiogenic shock • other relative contraindications to β-Blockade (PR interval > 0.24 s, II°- or III°- heart block, active asthma, or reactive airway disease)
ACE inhibitors	Class I	Orally within 24 h in patients with anterior MI, HF, EF < 0.40
	Class IIa	All patients
	Class III	An IV ACE inhibitor should not be given to patients within the first 24 hours of STEMI because of the risk of hypotension
ARB	Class I	Intolerant of ACE inhibitors, CHF or EF < 0.40
Nitrates	Class I	• First 48 h for persistent ischemia, HF, hypertension • After 48 hour for ischemia, heart failure
	Class III	Systolic BP < 90 mm Hg; Heart rate < 50 or > 100 beats per min
Magnesium	Class IIa	Hypomagnesemia, *torsades de pointes*
	Class III	Routine administration
Ca channel blockers	Class IIa	Verapamil or diltiazem if β-Blockers are ineffective or CI
	Class III	HF, LV dysfunction; immediate-release nifedipine

Class I indicates that procedure/treatment should be performed/administered;
Class IIa, it is reasonable to perform procedure/administer treatment;
Class IIb, procedure/treatment may be considered;
Class III, procedure/treatment should not be performed/administered because it is not helpful and may be harmful.

ACE = angiotensin converting enzyme; AF = atrial fibrillation; ARB = angiotensin-receptor blockers; ASA = aspirin; BP = blood pressure; CHF = congestive heart failure; CI = contraindications; DVT = deep venous thrombosis; F = ejection fraction; HF = heart failure; LMWH = low molecular weight heparin; LV = left ventricular; MI = myocardial infarction; PCI, = percutaneous coronary intervention; RV = right ventricular; Sx = symptoms; UFH = unfractionated heparin

3.4.6   Management of Acute Pulmonary Edema or Cardiogenic Shock

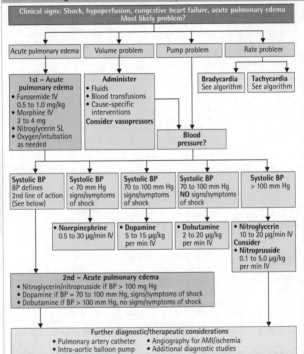

Reprinted from the Journal of the American College of Cardiology , Antman EM et al., ACC/AHA Guidelines for the Management of Patients With ST-Elevation Myocardial Infarction, e1–e211. Copyright 2004, with permission from the American College of Cardiology Foundation and the American Heart Association, Inc. Published by Elsevier Inc.

3.4.7 Long-term Therapy after ACS (UA/NSTEMI or STEMI)

Therapy Lifestyle	Goal
Smoking	Complete cessation, no exposure to environmental tobacco smoke
Blood pressure	Less than 140/90 mm Hg or < 130/80 mmHg if patient has diabetes or chronic kidney disease
Lipids	LDL-C substantially < 100 mg/dL, LDL preferably < 70 mg/dL; (If triglycerides are ≥ 200 mg/dL, non-HDL-C should be < 130 mg/dL
Physical activity	30 minutes, 7 days per week (minimum 5 days per week)
Body weight	BMI: 18.5 to 24.9 kg/m² Waist circumference: Men < 40 inches (102 cm), women < 35 inches (89 cm)
Diabetes	HbA$_{1c}$ < 7%

Pharmacotherapies	
Aspirin	For all stented patients without aspirin resistance, allergy, or increased risk of bleeding, aspirin 162 mg to 325 mg daily should be given for at least 1 month after bare metal stent implantation, 3 months after sirolimus-eluting stent implantation, and 6 months after paclitaxel-eluting stent implantation, after which long-term aspirin use should be continued indefinitely at a dose of 75 mg to 162 mg daily
Clopidogrel	For all post-PCI patients who receive a drug eluting stent (DES), clopidogrel 75 mg daily should be given for at least 12 months if patients are not at high risk of bleeding. For post-PCI patients receiving a bare metal stent, clopidogrel should be given for a minimum of 1 month and ideally up to 12 months (unless the patient is at increased risk of bleeding; then it should be given for a minimum of 2 weeks). For all STEMI patients not undergoing stenting (medical therapy alone or PTCA without stenting), treatment with clopidogrel should continue for at least 14 days and up to a year
Warfarin	In patients requiring warfarin, clopidogrel, and aspirin therapy, an INR of 2.0 to 2.5 is recommended with low dose aspirin (75 mg to 81 mg) and a 75 mg dose of clopidogrel
ACE inhibitors	ACE inhibitors should be started and continued indefinitely in all patients recovering from STEMI with LVEF less than or equal to 40% and for those with hypertension, diabetes, or chronic kidney disease, unless contraindicated

ARB	Use of angiotensin-receptor blockers is recommended in patients who are intolerant of ACE inhibitors and have HF or have had an MI with LVEF less than or equal to 40%.
Aldosterone blocker	Use of aldosterone blockade in post-MI patients without significant renal dysfunction or hyperkalemia is recommended in patients who are already receiving therapeutic doses of an ACE inhibitor and β-Blocker, have an LVEF of less than or equal to 40%, and have either diabetes or HF
β-Blockers	It is beneficial to start and continue β-Blocker therapy indefinitely in all patients who have had MI, acute coronary syndrome, or LV dysfunction with or without HF symptoms, unless contraindicated
Influenza vaccine	Patients with cardiovascular disease should have an annual influenza vaccination

3.5   Microvascular Angiopathy

3.5.1   Hypertension: General data

Causes of Hypertension
Essential: 90 %
No known cause
Secondary: 10 %
Sleep apnea
Chronic renal disease
Renovascular disease
Drugs
Cushing syndrome/steroids
Pheochromocytoma
Coarctation of aorta
Thyroid/parathyroid disease
Obstructive uropathy
Primary aldosteronism

Blood Pressure Classification JNC 7 2004		
JNC 7 Category	Systolic BP (mm Hg)	Diastolic BP (mm Hg)
Normal	< 120	< 80
Pre-hypertension	120–139	or 80–89
Hypertension, Stage I	140–159	or 90–99
Hypertension, Stage II	≥ 140	or ≥ 100
Isolated systolic HTN	> 140	< 90
Hypertensive urgency (no target organ damage)	High Stage II BP + symptoms	Sx: Headache, SOB, epistaxis, anxiety
Hypertensive emergency (with acutely progressive target organ damage)	> 180	> 120
Sx = Symptoms; SOB = shortness of breath		

Pathophysiology

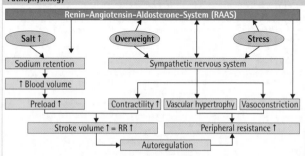

Cardiovascular Disease (CVD) Risk Factors JNC 7

- Hypertension
- Age: M > 55 y, F > 65 y
- Diabetes mellitus (DM)
- Smoking
- Dyslipidemia

- Metabolic syndrome
- Obesity: BMI ≥ 30 kg/m^2
- Physical inactivity
- Microalbuminuria or GFR < 60 mL/min
- Family history of premature CVD
  (M < 55 y, F < 65 y)

Goals of Treating Hypertension

- Blood pressure < 140/90 mm Hg (< 130/80 mm Hg if DM or chronic renal disease)
- Reduce target organ damage, cardiovascular and renal morbidity and mortality
- Significantly ↓ risk of stroke, MI, end-stage renal disease, and HF (average > 50% reduction)
- Stage I HTN with risk factors for CVD treated over 10 y prevents 1 death for every 11 patients (prevents 1 death for every 9 if target organ damage or CVD present) per JNC 7

Evaluation of Uncomplicated Hypertension

- History and physical incl BP measurement in both arms, sitting and standing
- Complete blood count, K, fasting blood sugar, Creatinine (Cr), Ca, lipid panel, urine analysis, ECG
- Consider urinary albumin/creatinine ratio
- Additional tests if onset < 30 yrs or > 60 yrs; hx sudden onset, severe, resistant, or paroxysmal HTN; abdominal trauma, mass, or bruit; abnormal urine analysis or elevated Cr; Cushing syndrome; target organ damage, or hypertensive emergency

Evaluation for Target Organ Damage

Vasculature

Ultrasound	
• Carotid plaques • Aortic aneurysm	• Vessel plaques: predictor for stroke or MI • Common carotid intimal-medial thickness ≥ 0.9 mm pathological

Eyes

Fundoscopy: Stages of hypertensive retinopathy	• I: Arteriolar constriction, ↓ arteriole/venule caliber ratio • II: Arteriovenous nicking and narrowing, "copper wiring" • III: Retinal hemorrhages, hard exudates, cotton-wool spots • IV: Bilateral papilledema

Heart — Abnormalities Associated with Hypertension

Electrocardiogram	• Sokolow-Lyon, Cornell Index voltage criterion for LVH • LVH with strain • Ischemia or prior MI • Arrhythmias; atrial fibrillation (common), PVCs, ventricular tachycardia ⇒ independent predictors for ↑ CV risk

Echocardiography 2D with Doppler flow
• LVH
• Heart Failure:
  - Stage A (NYHA class I): High risk for HF; no overt LV dysfunction/symptoms
  - Stage B (NYHA class I): EF < 40 %; asymptomatic
  - Stage C (NYHA class II-III): Symptomatic LV dysfunction
  - Stage D (NYHA class IV): End-stage HF; Sx at rest
	• LVH: Left ventricular mass index (LVMI) increased >102 gm/m² body surface area in men (or > 88 gm/m² body surface area in women)
	• Normal relative wall thickness (RWT): < 0.45
	• LV remodeling: normal LVMI + RWT > 0.45
	• Eccentric vs. concentric hypertrophy
	  Eccentric LVH: LVH + RWT < 0.45
	  Concentric LVH: LVH + RWT > 0.45
	• Interventricular septal hypertrophy, posterior wall thickened
	• LV diastolic dysfunction: normal contractility and EF, but compromised relaxation
	• LV systolic dysfunction: impaired contractility, low EF
	• E/F slope reduced
	• Left atrial enlargement

Kidneys

Chronic renal insufficiency Chronic renal failure	GFR < 60 ml/min; ↑ Cr > 1.5 mg/dL (men), > 1.3 mg/dL (women), elevated BUN, Cr, phosphate, K⁺; acidosis, anemia, low Ca⁺⁺, salt/water retention, bone disease, reduced eGFR
Proteinuria • estimatedGFR vs 24 h urine Cr clearance • Random spot urine • Albumin/Cr ratio	• Microalbuminuria: 30–300 mg / 24 h (20–200 mg/g Cr on spot urine) ⇒ predictor for ↑ risk CVD; nephropathy • Macroalbuminuria: > 300 mg / 24 h (> 200 mg/g Cr on spot urine) ⇒ renal parenchymal disease
End stage renal disease	• Inadequate Dx and Tx ⇒ ESRD resulting from HTN is rising • GFR < 10; systemic disease; dialysis / renal transplant

Brain

MRI CT scan	• Consider MRI if microinfarctions suspected, or dementia • Consider CT r/o acute bleed
Cognitive function tests	Frequent serial testing demonstrates early cognitive deficits

DM = diabetes mellitus, BUN = blood urea nitrogen, Cr = creatinine, CT = computer tomography, CVD = cardiovascular disease, Dx = Diagnosis, ESRD = end stage renal disease, GFR = glomerular filtration rate, HTN = Hypertension, LVH = left ventricular hypertrophy, MI = myocardial infarction, MRI = magnetic resonance imaging, NYHA = New York Heart Association, r/o = rule out, Sx = Symptoms

Lifestyle Modifications for Patients

1. Weight reduction if overweight	6. Monitor blood pressure regularly
2. Adopt DASH eating plan and lifestyle	7. Reduce dietary sodium
3. Eat 5 servings fresh fruits/vegetables; low-fat dairy; diet high in Ca++, K+ and low in fat, cholesterol, Na+	8. Regular aerobic exercise (per physician's approval) 30 min/day most days
4. Alcohol in moderation	9. Rest, relaxation, stress reduction
5. Take medications as prescribed	10. Smoking cessation

Lifestyle Modifications to Manage Hypertension JNC 7, Table 9

Modification	SBP Reduction	Considerations
Weight loss (maintain BMI 18.5–24.9 kg/m²)	5–20 mm Hg/ 10 kg	Weight loss of even 10 lbs may reduce BP in obese patient
Limit alcohol consumption (M 1 oz, F ½ oz per day)	2–4 mm Hg	Heavy alcohol ↑ BP and ↑ LV mass
Regular aerobic exercise (30 min/day most days)	4–9 mm Hg	Advise medical clearance before initiating if CVD risk
Reduce dietary sodium (< 2.4 g Na or 6 g NaCl)	2–8 mm Hg	Most effective if low renin levels
DASH diet	8–14 mm Hg	Adopt diet rich in vegetables, fruits, and low-fat dairy; low in cholesterol, saturated and total fat, and high in K+ and Ca++

Causes of Resistant Hypertension

Non-compliance
Improper measurement of BP
Volume overload and pseudotolerance
- Sodium intake excessive
- Renal disease with volume retension

Treatment-related
- Inadequate drug dosage
- Inadequate treatment with diuretics
- Irrational combination therapy (dosing interval exceeds half-life, or prescriptions with same mechanism of action)

Drug-induced causes
- Sympathomimetics
- Appetite suppressants/anorectics
- Oral contraceptives
- Licorice
- NSAID
- Antidepressants
- Erythropoietin
- Steroids
- Cocaine, amphetamines, stimulants
- Over-the-counter (OTC) drugs and herbal preparations

Associated conditions	Other causes of acute hypertension
• Weight gain, obesity	• Delirium tremens
• Excessive alcohol, alcoholism	• MAO inhibitor + tyramine or TCA
• Chronic pain	• Serotonin syndrome
• Organic brain syndrome	• Neuroleptic malignant syndrome
• Sleep apnea	• Malignant hyperthermia /heat stroke
• Acute illness	• Thyroid storm
• Lupus, vasculitides	• Acute angle-closure glaucoma
• Other; complete medical history essential	• CNS pathology, trauma

Resistant hypertension: failure to achieve BP control on 2 drugs + diuretic.; TCA = tricyclic antidepressant

Compelling Indications for Individual Drug Classes (JNC 7)

Recommended Drugs
1 = consider first-line
2 = consider adding, or use as alternative choice
3 = consider adding, or use as second-line choice

Compelling Indications	Diuretic	β-Blocker (BB)	Ca-Antagonist	ACE Inhibitor	Angiotensin-Rec-Ant. (ARB)	Aldosterone Antagonist	α₁-Blocker	Clonidine (α₂-Agonist)	α-Methyldopa	Hydralazine
Uncomplicated hypertension	1	2	2	2	2					
Hypertensive urgency*		αβ*		1*			1*	1		
Geriatric patient > 65 yrs	1	1	2	1	2					
LV Hypertrophy	1	2	2	1	1					
HF: Stage A NYHA Class I	1			1	2					
HF: Stage B NYHA Class I LVEF < 40%		1		1	2					
HF: Stage C NYHA Class II-III	loop	1		1	2	1				
HF: Stage D NYHA Class IV Stage C rx plus inotropes + interventions	loop	1		1	2	1				
High risk of Cardiovascular Disease	1	1	1	1						
Ischemic heart dz, stable angina		1	2							
Post-Myocardial infarction (MI)		1		1		1				
Prevent recurrent stroke	1			1						

Compelling Indications for Individual Drug Classes (JNC 7)

Recommended Drugs
1 = consider first-line
2 = consider adding, or use as alternative choice
3 = consider adding, or use as second-line choice

Compelling Indications	Diuretic	β-Blocker (BB)	Ca-Antagonist	ACE Inhibitor	Angiotensin-Rec.-Ant. (ARB)	Aldosterone Antagonist	α_1-Blocker	Clonidine (α_2-Agonist)	α-Methyldopa	Hydralazine
Chronic kidney disease	Cr >2.5 loop			1	1					
Diabetes mellitus (DM), type 1 or 2	2	2	3	1	2					
DM with microalbuminemia	2	2	3	1	1					
Hyperuricemia	avd thia									
Benign prostatic hypertrophy							1			
Pregnancy		2**	3	avd	avd				1	ecla

Diuretics: Start with thiazide unless otherwise indicated. BB: use with caution in DM. Ca-channel-blockers (CCB): Long-acting dihydropyridine or nondihydropyridine (short-acting CCBs not recommended). Hypertensive urgency*: Cautious use of shorter-acting oral drugs monitored in acute care setting eg. $\alpha\beta$* labetalol (combined α–β-Blocker),1*captopril (+/– loop), prazocin, clonidine. Pregnancy**: Labetalol ($\alpha\beta$) is a ↑ popular alternative to methyldopa. Some BB are implicated in IUGR; avd = avoid; BB = β-Blockers; ecla = eclampsie; IUGR = intrauterine fetal growth retardation; loop = loop diuretic; thia = thiazide

Highlights JNC 7 on Prevention, Detection, Evaluation, and Therapy of Hypertension

- If > 50 y, SBP > 140 mm Hg is a greater risk factor for CVD than diastolic BP.
- **Risk of CVD doubles** for every 20/10 mm Hg above 115/75 mm Hg.
- **Non-pharmacologic therapy (lifestyle modification)** is recommended for pre-hypertension, and for all stages of hypertension.
- **Thiazide**-type diuretics are first line treatment for most people with uncomplicated HTN (alone or in combination). Most patients will require two or more antihypertensives.
- High risk comorbidities with **compelling indications,** the presence of **target organ damage,** or **BP > 20/10 mm Hg above goal** may direct strategy for **combination therapy.**
- A trusting **doctor–patient relationship,** patient **motivation** and the **physician's judgment** about patient management are most important and are ultimately responsible.
- **Note:** Monotherapy is often not effective alone to achieve BP 140/90 (130/80 mmHg if DM or chronic kidney disease). Fixed-dose combinations simplify therapy and may be cost-effective.

JNC = The Seventh Report of the Joint National Committee on Prevention, Detection, Evaluation, and Treatment of High Blood Pressure, US Dept Health and Human Services, NIH, 2004

3.5.2 Hypertensive Crisis – Definition and Terms

It is the clinical state of the patient and the degree and progression of target organ damage that defines a hypertensive emergency and not the absolute level of blood pressure.

Definition		Management
Hypertensive urgency	• Marked elevations of BP, usually higher than 180/110 mm Hg. • Evidence of target organ damage is often present, but is nonprogressive. • Symptoms may include headache, shortness of breath, and pedal edema	Management in the emergency department with oral agents is reasonable, depending on the individual's presentation, and follow-up within 24 to 48 hours is recommended
Hypertensive emergency	• Severe elevation in BP > 180/120 mm Hg, and often higher than 220/140 mm Hg, complicated by clinical evidence of progressive target organ dysfunction. • Examples are hypertensive ence-phalopathy, intracranial hemor-rhage, acute MI, acute LV failure, dissecting aneurysm, acute renal failure, and eclampsia of pregnancy.	Patients require immediate admission and BP reduction (not to normal ranges) to prevent or limit further target organ damage

Pharmacologic Treatment of Hypertensive Emergencies					
Drug	Dose	Mechanism	Onset	Duration	Side effects
Sodium nitroprusside	0.25–10 µg/kg/min as IV infusion	Arterial dilator and venodilator	Imme-diate	2–3 min after infusion	Nausea, vomiting; prolonged use may cause thiocyanate intoxication, methemoglobin-emia, acidosis, cyanide poisoning; bags, bottles, delivery sets must be light resistant
Nitroglycerin	5–100 µg as IV infusion	Venodilator	2–5 min	5–10 min	Headache, tachy-cardia, flushing, requires special delivery system because of drug binding to PVC tubing
Nicardipine	5–15 mg/h as IV infusion	Dihydro-pyridine calcium channel blocker	1–5 min	15–30 min, but may exceed 12 h after prolonged infusion	Tachycardia, nausea, vomiting, headache, increased intracranial pres-sure; hypotension may be protracted after prolonged infusions
Hydralazine	5–20 mg as IV bolus or 10–40 mg IM; repeat every 4–6 h	Arterial dilator	10 min IV 20–30 min IM	1 h (IV); 4–6 h (IM)	Tachycardia, headache, vomiting, aggravation of angina pectoris, sodium and water retention, increased intracranial pressure
Enalaprilat	0.625–1.25 mg every 6 h as IV injection	ACE inhibitor	Within 30 min	12–24 h	Renal failure in pa-tients with bilateral renal artery stenosis, hypotension

Esmolol	500–μg/kg bolus injection IV or 50–300 μg/kg/min by infusion	β-Blocker	1–5 min	15–30 min	First-degree heart block, congestive heart failure, asthma
Labetalol	20–40 mg as IV bolus every 10 min; up to 2 mg/min as IV infusion	β-Blocker	5–10 min	2–6 h	Bronchoconstriction, heart block, orthostatic hypotension, bradycardia
Phento-lamine	5–10 mg as IV bolus	α-Blocker	1–2 min	10–30 min	Tachycardia, orthostatic hypotension

3.5.3 Hypertensive Heart Disease

Recommendations regarding blood pressure target and specific drug indications in selected population with ischemic heart disease (IHD) or those at risk for IHD.

Area of Concern	Target BP (mm Hg)	Lifestyle Modification[1]	Specific drug interactions	Comments
General CAD prevention	< 140/90	Yes	Any effective antihypertensive drug or combination[1]	If SBP ≥ 160 mm Hg or DBP ≥ 100 mm Hg, then start with 2 drugs
High CAD risk[2]	< 130/80	Yes	ACEI or ARB or CCB or thiazide diuretic or combination	If SBP ≥ 160 mm Hg or DBP ≥ 100 mm Hg, then start with 2 drugs
Stable angina	< 130/80	Yes	β-Blocker and ACEI or ARB	If β-Blocker contraindicated, or if side effects occur, can substitute diltiazem or verapamil (but not if bradycardia or LVD is present)
				Can add dihydropyridine CCB (not diltiazem or verapamil) to β-Blocker
				A thiazide diuretic can be added for BP control

Area of Concern	Target BP (mm Hg)	Lifestyle Modification[1]	Secific drug interactions	Comments
UA/NSTEMI	< 130/80	Yes	β-Blocker (if patient is hemodynamically stable) *and* ACEI or ARB[3]	If β-Blocker contraindicated, or if side effects occur, can substitute diltiazem or verapamil (but not if bradycardia or LVD is present)
				Can add dihydropyridine CCB (not diltiazem or verapamil) to β-Blocker
				A thiazide diuretic can be added for BP control
STEMI	< 130/80	Yes	β-Blocker (if patient is hemodynamically stable) *and* ACEI or ARB[4]	If Betablocker contraindicated, or if side effects occur, can substitute diltiazem or verapamil (but not if bradycardia or LVD is present)
				Can add dihydropyridine CCB (not diltiazem or verapamil) to β-Blocker
				A thiazide diuretic can be added for BP control
LVD	< 120/80	Yes	ACEI or ARB *and* β-Blocker *and* aldosterone antagonist[5] *and* thiazide or loop diuretic *and* hydralazine/isosorbide dinitrate (blacks)	Contraindicated: verapamil, diltiazem, clonidine, moxonidine, α-Blockers

ACEI = angiotensin converting enzyme inhibitor, ARB = angiotensin receptor blocker, CAD = coronary artery disease, CCB = calcium channel blocker, DBP = diastolic blood pressure, HF = Heart failure, LVD = left ventricular dysfunction, NSTEMI = non-ST-segment elevation myocardial infarction, SBP = systolic blood pressure, UA = unstable angina; [1]Weight loss if appropriate, healthy diet (including sodium restriction), exercise, smoking cessation, and alcohol moderation; [2]Diabetes mellitus, chronic kidney disease, known CAD or CAD equivalent (carotid artery disease, peripheral arterial disease, abdominal aortic aneurysm), or 10-year Framingham risk score > 10%, [3]Evidence supports ACEI (or ARB), CCB, or thiazide diuretic as first-line therapy; [4]If anterior MI is present, if hypertension persists, if LV dysfunction or HF is present, or if the patient has diabetes mellitus; [5]If severe HF is present (NYHA III or IV, or LVEF < 40 % and clinical HF);

3.5.4 Diabetic Heart Disease

Epidemiology

- The prevalence of diabetes mellitus is rapidly increasing in both developing and developed countries
- CHD is highly prevalent and is the major cause of morbidity and mortality in diabetic patients.
- Patients with CHD and prediabetic states should undergo lifestyle modifications aimed at preventing DM
- Among patients with CHD and DM, routine use of aspirin and an ACE inhibitor is recommended unless contraindicated or not tolerated and optimal glycemic, blood pressure, and lipid control are strongly recommended.
- For blood pressure control in DM, ACE inhibitor and ARBs are considered as first-line therapy

Components of a Comprehensive Diabetes Evaluation

Medical History

- Age and characteristics of onset of diabetes (e.g., diabetic ketoacidosis (DKA), asymptomatic laboratory finding)
- Eating patterns, physical activity habits, nutritional status, and weight history; growth and development in children and adolescents
- Diabetes education history
- Review of previous treatment regimens and response to therapy (HbA$_{1C}$ records)

Current Treatment of Diabetes, Including Medications, Meal Plan, Physical Activity Patterns and Results of Glucose Monitoring, and Patient's Use of Data

- DKA frequency, severity, and cause
- Hypoglycemic episodes
  - Hypoglycemia awareness
  - Any severe hypoglycemia: frequency and cause
- History of diabetes-related complications
  - Microvascular: retinopathy, nephropathy, neuropathy (sensory, including history of foot lesions; autonomic, including sexual dysfunction and gastroparesis)
  - Macrovascular: CHD, cerebrovascular disease, peripheral artery disease (PAD)
  - Other: psychosocial problems*, dental disease*

Physical Examination

- Height, weight, BMI
- Blood pressure determination, including orthostatic measurements when indicated
- Fundoscopic examination*
- Thyroid palpation
- Skin examination (for acanthosis nigricans and insulin injection sites)
- Comprehensive foot examination:
  - Inspection
  - Palpation of dorsalis pedis and posterior tibial pulses
  - Presence/absence of patellar and Achilles reflexes
  - Determination of proprioception, vibration, and monofilament sensation

Laboratory Evaluation

- HbA$_{1C}$, if results not available within past 2-3 months
- If not performed/available within past year:
  - Fasting lipid profile, including total, LDL- and HDL cholesterol and triglycerides
  - Liver function tests
  - Test for urine albumin excretion with spot urine albumin/creatinine ratio
  - Serum creatinine and calculated GFR
  - TSH in type 1 diabetes, dyslipidemia, or women over age 50 years

Referrals

- Annual dilated eye exam
- Family planning for women of reproductive age
- Registered dietitian for Medical Nutrition Therapy (MNT)
- Diabetes Self Management Education (DSME)
- Dental examination
- Mental health professional, if needed

* See appropriate referrals for these categories.
Copyright 2010 American Diabetes Association. From Diabetes Care, Vol. 33, 2010; S11–S61.
Reproduced by permission of The American Diabetes Association.

Summary of Recommendations for Glycemic, Blood Pressure, and Lipid Control for Adults with Diabetes

- HbA$_{1C}$ < 7.0%*
- Blood pressure < 130/80 mmHg
- Lipids: LDL cholesterol < 100 mg/dL (< 2.6 mmol/L)**

*Referenced to a nondiabetic range of 4.0–6.0% using a DCCT-based assay. **In individuals with overt CVD, a lower LDL cholesterol goal of 70 mg/dL (1.8 mmol/L), using a high dose of a statin, is an option.
Copyright 2010 American Diabetes Association. From Diabetes Care, Vol. 33, 2010; S11–S61.
Reproduced by permission of The American Diabetes Association.

Diabetes and CHD and Optimal Therapy

- Consider aspirin therapy (75-162 mg/ day) as a primary prevention strategy in those with type 1 or type 2 diabetes at increased cardiovascular risk (10-year risk >10%). This includes most men > 50 years of age or women > 60 years of age who have at least one additional major risk factor (family history of CHD, hypertension, smoking, dyslipidemia, or albuminuria)
- Use aspirin therapy (75-162 mg/day) as a secondary prevention strategy in those with diabetes with CHD
- Combination therapy with aspirin (75-162 mg/day) and clopidogrel (75 mg/day) is reasonable for up to a year after an acute coronary syndrome
- Patients with a systolic blood pressure 130-139 mm Hg or a diastolic blood pressure 80-89 mm Hg may be given lifestyle therapy alone for a maximum of 3 months, and then if targets are not achieved, patients should be treated with the addition of pharmacological agents
- Pharmacologic therapy for patients with diabetes and hypertension should be paired with a regimen that includes either an ACE inhibitor or an angiotensin II-receptor blocker (ARB)
- In individuals without overt CVD, the primary goal is an LDL cholesterol < 100 mg/dL (2.6 mmol/L) and in individuals with overt CVD, a lower LDL cholesterol goal of < 70 mg/dL (1.8 mmol/L), using a high dose of a statin, is an option
- Include smoking cessation counseling as a routine component of diabetes care
- In asymptomatic CHD patients, evaluate risk factors to stratify patients by 10-year risk, and treat risk factors accordingly
- In patients with known CHD, ACE inhibitor, aspirin, and statin therapy (if not contraindicated) should be routinely used to reduce the risk of future cardiovascular events
- In patients with a prior MI, β-Blockers should be continued for at least 2 years after the event
- Avoid thiazolidinedione (TZD) treatment in patients with symptomatic heart failure
- Metformin may be used in patients with stable HF if renal function is normal. It should be avoided in unstable or hospitalized patients with HF

3.6 Inflammatory Heart and Vascular Diseases

3.6.1 Myocarditis

Epidemiology

- Myocarditis is an inflammatory disease of the myocardium with a wide range of clinical presentations.
- Diagnosis is based on established histologic, immunologic, and immunochemical criteria.
- Myocarditis is defined as an inflammatory infiltrate of the myocardium with necrosis and/or degeneration of adjacent myocytes.
- The condition usually manifests in an otherwise healthy person and can result in rapidly progressive (and often fatal) heart failure and arrhythmia.
- Myocarditis is caused by a wide variety of infectious organisms, autoimmune disorders, and exogenous agents, with genetic and environmental predisposition.

Clinicopathological Classification

- **Fulminant myocarditis** - Typically follows a viral prodrome with distinct onset of illness comprising severe cardiovascular compromise with ventricular dysfunction and multiple foci of active myocarditis; either resolves spontaneously or results in death
- **Acute myocarditis** - Has a less distinct onset of illness, with established ventricular dysfunction and may progress to dilated cardiomyopathy
- **Chronic active myocarditis** - A less distinct onset of illness, with clinical and histologic relapses, development of ventricular dysfunction associated with chronic inflammatory changes (including giant cells on histopathology)
- **Chronic persistent myocarditis** - Less distinct onset of illness; persistent histologic infiltrate with foci of myocyte necrosis without ventricular dysfunction despite symptoms (e.g., chest pain, palpitations)

Causes

Viral	Enterovirus, coxsackie B, adenovirus, influenza, cytomegalovirus, Epstein-Barr virus, HIV-1, mumps, rubeola, varicella, variola/vaccinia, arbovirus, respiratory syncytial virus, herpes simplex virus, rabies, parvovirus
Rickettsial	Scrub typhus, Rocky Mountain Spotted Fever, Q fever
Bacterial	Diphtheria, tuberculosis, streptococci, meningococci, brucellosis, clostridia, staphylococci, melioidosis, *Mycoplasma pneumoniae*, psittacosis
Spirochetal	Syphilis, leptospirosis/Weil disease, relapsing fever/Borrelia, Lyme disease
Fungal	Candidiasis, aspergillosis, cryptococcosis, histoplasmosis, actinomycosis, blastomycosis, coccidioidomycosis, mucormycosis
Protozoal	Chagas disease, toxoplasmosis, trypanosomiasis, malaria, leishmaniasis, balantidiasis, sarcosporidiosis

Helminthic	Trichinosis, echinococcosis, schistosomiasis, heterophyiasis, cysticercosis, visceral larva migrans, filariasis
Bites/stings	Scorpion, snake, black widow spider, wasp venom, tick paralysis
Drugs	• Chemotherapeutic drugs - Doxorubicin and anthracyclines, streptomycin, cyclophosphamide, interleukin-2, anti-HER-2 receptor antibody/herceptin • Antibiotics - penicillin, chloramphenicol, sulfonamides • Antihypertensive drugs - methyldopa, spironolactone • Antiseizure drugs - phenytoin, carbamazepine • Amphetamines, cocaine, catecholamines
Chemicals	Hydrocarbons, carbon monoxide, arsenic, lead, phosphorus, mercury, cobalt
Acute rheumatic fever	
Systemic inflammatory disease	Giant cell myocarditis, sarcoidosis, Kawasaki disease, Crohn disease, systemic lupus erythematosus, ulcerative colitis, Wegener granulomatosis, thyrotoxicosis, scleroderma, rheumatoid arthritis
Diagnosis	
History	• Chest pain, dyspnea, orthopnea, paroxysmal nocturnal dyspnea (PND) • Patients may present with mild symptoms of chest pain, fever, sweats, chills, and dyspnea. • In post-viral myocarditis, patients may present with a history of recent flulike syndrome of fevers, arthralgias, and malaise or pharyngitis, tonsillitis, or upper respiratory tract infection. • Symptoms of palpitations, syncope, or even sudden cardiac death may develop, due to underlying ventricular arrhythmias or atrioventricular block (especially in giant cell myocarditis)
Physical examination	
Acute heart failure	Patients with myocarditis usually present with signs and symptoms of acute decompensated heart failure (e.g., tachycardia, gallop, pulmonary edema) and pericardial rub in those with concomitant pericarditis
Arrhythmias	Sustained ventricular tachycardia and rapidly progressive heart failure is seen in giant cell myocarditis

Diagnostic Tests	
Laboratory investigations	Elevated cardiac enzymes is seen in at least 50% of patients with biopsy-proven myocarditis
ECG	Usually shows nonspecific changes e.g., sinus tachycardia, nonspecific ST- or T-wave changes
Echocardiography	Performed to assess left ventricular systolic function and exclude other causes of heart failure (e.g., valvular, congenital)
MRI	Gadolinium-enhanced magnetic resonance imaging (MRI) is used for assessment of the extent of inflammation and cellular edema
Endomyocardial biopsy	Endomyocardial biopsy (EMB) is the gold standard for diagnosis of myocarditis, although it has limited sensitivity and specificity, because inflammation can be diffuse or focal. Histologic diagnosis seldom has an impact on therapeutic strategies except in cases of giant cell myocarditis. The risk of adverse events includes 0.5% probability of perforation.

Treatment	
Withdrawal of the offending agent	• Indicated based on the clinical situation (e.g., cardiotoxic drugs, alcohol, etc). • Nonsteroidal anti-inflammatory agents should be avoided in the acute phase, because their use may interfere with myocardial healing.
Immunosuppression	Empirical treatment with immunosuppression for systemic autoimmune disease, especially in giant cell myocarditis and sarcoid myocarditis, is often given
Supportive therapy	For symptoms of acute heart failure, use of diuretics, vasodilators, and angiotensin-converting enzyme (ACE) is indicated
Inotropic drugs	E.g., dobutamine, milrinone may be necessary for severe decompensation, although they are highly arrhythmogenic
Long term treatment	Follows the same medical regimen, including ACE inhibitors, β-Blockers, and aldosterone-receptor antagonists
Intra-aortic balloon pump (ABP) and Left ventricular assistive devices (LVADs) and extracorporeal membrane oxygenation	May be indicated for short-term circulatory support if needed for cardiogenic shock.

3.6.2 Endocarditis

Epidemiology

- Infective endocarditis (IE) is an infection of the endocardial surface of the heart.
- The incidence of IE is approximately 2-4 cases per 100 000 persons per year.
- IE produces a wide variety of systemic signs and symptoms through several mechanisms, including both sterile and infected emboli and various immunological phenomena.
- In the last two decades, the clinical characteristics of IE have changed significantly
- Cases of nosocomial infective endocarditis (NIE), intravenous drug abuse (IVDA) IE, and prosthetic valve endocarditis (PVE) have significantly increased.
- Libman-Sacks endocarditis (otherwise known as verrucous, marantic, or nonbacterial thrombotic endocarditis) is the most characteristic cardiac manifestation of the autoimmune disease systemic lupus erythematosus.

Causes

- *Staphylococcus aureus* is the most common cause of acute IE, including PVE and IVDA IE.
- *Streptococcus viridans* accounts for approximately 50-60% of cases of subacute disease.
- *Streptococcus intermedius* group may be acute or subacute and accounts for 15% of streptococcal IE cases.
- *Abiotrophia* species (formerly known as nutritionally variant streptococci) account for approximately 5% of subacute cases of IE.
- Group D streptococci cases are subacute and source is the gastrointestinal or genitourinary tract.
- Nonenterococcal group D organisms infection often reflects underlying abnormalities of the large bowel (e.g., ulcerative colitis, polyps, cancer).
- Group B streptococci disease develops in pregnant patients and older patients with underlying diseases (e.g., cancer, diabetes, alcoholism).
- Group A, C, and G streptococci
- Coagulase-negative S aureus causes subacute disease.
- *Pseudomonas aeruginosa* IE is usually acute, except when it involves the right side of the heart in IVDA IE.
- HACEK organisms (i.e., *Haemophilus aphrophilus*, *Actinobacillus actinomycetemcomitans*, *Cardiobacterium hominis*, *Eikenella corrodens*, *Kingella kingae*) organisms usually cause subacute disease and account for approximately 5% of IE cases.
- Fungi usually cause subacute disease. The most common organism of both fungal NVE and fungal PVE is *Candida albicans*. Fungal IVDA IE is usually caused by *Candida parapsilosis* or *Candida tropicalis*.
- Bartonella species IE typically develops in homeless males who have extremely substandard hygiene. Bartonella must be considered in cases of culture-negative endocarditis among homeless individuals.
- Polymicrobial infective endocarditis is observed in cases of IVDA IE

Duke Criteria	
Pathologic criteria	• Culture or histology directly from valve, after surgery or autopsy
Clinical criteria	(2 major criteria, or 1 major + 3 minor criteria, or 5 minor criteria)
Major criteria	• Positive blood cultures x 2 of typical organisms • Positive echocardiogram (vegetation, abscess, prosthetic valve, or dehiscence); or presence of new valvular regurgitation
Minor criteria	• Predisposition (IV drug abuse or cardiac abnormality) • Fever > 38°C • Embolic disease • Vascular/immunological signs (glomerulonephritis, Osler nodes) • Positive blood culture or echocardiogram that does not meet major criterion

Risk Stratification	
High-Risk	**Moderate-Risk**

• Prosthetic cardiac valve
• History of infective endocarditis
• Congenital heart disease (CHD)*
  - Unrepaired cyanotic CHD, including palliative shunts and conduits
  - Completely repaired congenital heart defect with prosthetic material or device, whether placed by surgery or by catheter intervention, during the first 6 months after the procedure
  - Repaired CHD with residual defects at the site or adjacent to the site of a prosthetic patch or prosthetic device (which inhibits endothelialization)
• Cardiac transplantation recipients with cardiac valvular disease
	• Acquired valvular heart disease
	• Mitral valve prolapse (MVP) with mitral regurgitation (MR) or thickened redundant leaflets
	• Most congenital heart diseases
	• Hypertrophic cardiomyopathy

*Except for the conditions listed above, antibiotic prophylaxis is no longer recommended for any other form of CHD

Prophylaxis	
Conditions Not Requiring Prophylaxis	
Isolated secundum ASD	6 months after repair of ASD, VSD, or PDA
Functional heart murmurs	MVP without MR or thickened or redundant leaflets
Previous CABG	Cardiac pacemakers or implanted defibrillators

Procedures Requiring Prophylaxis	
Procedure Type	**When Prophylaxis Is Needed**
Dental	High and moderate risk conditions; any procedures likely to cause bleeding
Respiratory tract	High and moderate risk conditions, tonsillectomy, adenoidectomy, procedures involving the respiratory mucosa, rigid brochoscopy
GI Tract	High risk conditions, optional for moderate risk conditions, sclerotherapy for varices, esophageal dilatation, ERCP with biliary obstruction, biliary tract surgery, procedures involving the intestinal mucosa
Genitourinary tract	High and moderate risk conditions, prostatic surgery, cystoscopy, urethral dilatation

Prophylaxis Regimen	
Treatment of Choice	**Alternative Treatment**
Dental, Upper Respiratory Tract, and Esophageal Procedures	
• amoxicillin PO 2 g, 1 hour before procedure OR • ampicillin IV/IM 2 g, 30 minutes before procedure	• clindamycin 600 mg PO/IV • clarithromycin 500 mg PO • azithromycin 500 mg PO • cephalexin or cefadroxil 2 g PO • cefazolin 1 g IM/IV
Urologic Procedures (Moderate-Risk Conditions)	
• amoxicillin PO or ampicillin IM/IV	• vancomycin 1 g IV over 1 ~ 2 hours
Urologic Procedures (High-Risk Conditions)	
• ampicillin 2 g IV/IM + gentamicin 1.5 mg/kg within 30 minutes of starting procedure. • 6 hours later, give ampicillin 1 g IV/IM or amoxicillin 1 g PO	• vancomycin 1 g IV + gentamicin 1.5 mg/kg IV/IM (not to exceed 120 mg)

3.6.3 Pericarditis

Epidemiology

- Acute pericarditis is an inflammation of the pericardium characterized by chest pain, pericardial friction rub, and serial electrocardiographic changes
- Acute pericarditis comprises approximately 1% of emergency room visits in patients with ST-segment elevation
- In most cases of acute pericarditis, the pericardium is acutely inflamed and has an infiltration of polymorphonuclear (PMN) leukocytes .

Causes	
Idiopathic	
Infection	
Viral	<ul><li>Most common cause of acute pericarditis and accounts for 1-10% of cases.</li><li>Causative viruses include coxsackievirus B, echovirus, adenoviruses, influenza A and B viruses, Enterovirus, mumps virus, Epstein-Barr virus, human immunodeficiency virus (HIV), herpes simplex virus type 1, varicella-zoster virus, measles virus, parainfluenza virus type 2, and respiratory syncytial virus, cytomegalovirus, hepatitis A, hepatitis B, and hepatitis C.</li><li>It is usually a self-limited disease that lasts 1-3 weeks.</li></ul>
Bacterial	<ul><li>This accounts for 1-8% of cases and causes purulent pericarditis.</li><li>Bacterial pericarditis develops from either direct pulmonary extension, hematogenous spread, myocardial abscess, or endocarditis</li><li>Organisms isolated include gram-positive species such as *Streptococcus pneumoniae* and other *Streptococcus* species and *Staphylococcus* and gram-negative species include *Proteus, Escherichia coli, Pseudomonas, Klebsiella, Salmonella, Shigella, Neisseria meningitidis,* and *Haemophilus influenzae.*</li><li>Less common organisms include *Legionella, Nocardia, Actinobacillus, Rickettsia, Borrelia burgdorferi* (Lyme borreliosis), *Listeria, Leptospira, Chlamydophila psittaci,* and *Treponema pallidum* (syphilis).</li></ul>

Tubercular	• Tuberculosis accounts for 2–4% of cases. • The diagnostic yield for acid-fast bacilli in pericardial fluid is fairly low (between 30% and 76%). • Pericardial biopsy has a much better yield (approximately 100%). • Elevated adenosine deaminase in pericardial fluid is useful for diagnosing tuberculosis. Studies note greater than 90% sensitivity and specificity with levels higher than 50–70 U/L. • The mortality rate approaches 50%.
Other infectious agents	• Fungal organisms include *Histoplasma, Blastomyces, Coccidioides, Aspergillus,* and *Candida.* • Parasitic organisms include *Entamoeba, Echinococcus,* and *Toxoplasma.*
Inflammatory disorders	• Rheumatoid arthritis • Ankylosing spondylitis • Systemic lupus erythematosus • Inflammatory bowel disease • Scleroderma • Wegener granulomatosis • Rheumatic fever • Vasculitis (e.g., giant cell arteritis, polyarteritis nodosa) • Sarcoidosis • Polymyositis • Sjögren syndrome • Behçet syndrome • Mixed connective-tissue disease • Whipple disease • Reiter syndrome • Familial Mediterranean fever • Serum sickness
Metabolic disorders	• Renal failure • Hypothyroidism
Cardiovascular diseases	• Post-Myocardial infarction • Aortic dissection
Neoplasm	Lung, mediastinal, etc.
Drugs	• Some medications, including penicillin and cromolyn sodium, induce pericarditis through a hypersensitivity reaction. • The anthracycline antineoplastic agents, such as doxorubicin and cyclophosphamide, have direct cardiac toxicity and can cause acute pericarditis and myocarditis. • Pericarditis can develop from a drug-induced SLE syndrome caused by medications including procainamide, hydralazine, methyldopa, isoniazid • Methysergide causes constrictive pericarditis through mediastinal fibrosis. • Dantrolene, phenytoin, and minoxidil produce pericarditis through an unknown mechanism.

Diagnosis	
History	• Chest pain, dyspnea, fever • Chest pain is the most common symptom. • The quality of the pain may be sharp, dull, aching, burning, or pressing. • Pain usually is precordial with referral to the trapezius ridge. • It is worse during inspiration, when lying flat, or during swallowing
Physical Examination	
Pericardial rub	• A pericardial friction rub is pathognomonic for acute pericarditis. • The rub has a scratching, grating sound similar to leather rubbing against leather. • Auscultation with the diaphragm of the stethoscope over the left lower sternal edge allows the best detection of the rub. • Auscultation during end-expiration with the patient sitting up and leaning forward increases the likelihood of hearing the rub • Typical rubs are triphasic. They are composed of (1) an atrial systolic rub that precedes S_1, (2) a ventricular systolic rub between S_1 and S_2 and coincident with the peak carotid pulse, and (3) an early diastolic rub after S_2 (usually the faintest).
Beck triad (eventually)	i.e., hypotension; jugular venous distention and muffled heart sounds may occur in patients with cardiac tamponade.
Diagnostic Tests	
Laboratory investigations	Elevated cardiac enzymes is seen in some patients with pericarditis and is related to concomitant myocarditis
Chest radiography	Usually normal in uncomplicated pericarditis. An enlarged cardiac silhouette may be the first indication of a large pericardial effusion
ECG	Shows characteristic serial changes: • **Stage 1:** diffuse concave upward ST-segment elevation without reciprocal ST-segment depression. Depression of PR segment is unique to pericarditis • **Stage 2:** ST-segment returns to baseline and T wave flattens • **Stage 3:** ST-segment is isoelectric, T wave inverts in leads II, AVF, and V_4-V_6 • **Stage 4:** Gradual resolution of T wave inversion
Echocardiography	Helpful if pericardial effusion is suspected on clinical or radiographic grounds, the illness lasts longer than 1 week, or myocarditis or purulent pericarditis is suspected.

Treatment

Treatment for specific causes	Directed according to the underlying cause
Aspirin	Recommended for treatment of pericarditis after myocardial infarction
Colchicine	Alone or in combination with an NSAID, can be considered for patients with recurrent or continued symptoms beyond 14 days.
Corticosteroids	Should not be used for initial treatment of pericarditis unless indicated for the underlying disease, the patient has no response to NSAIDs or colchicine, or both are contraindicated

3.6.4   Vasculitis

Epidemiology

- Vasculitis refers to inflammation of blood vessels
- Arteries and veins of any size in any organ may be affected, leading to ischemic damage to organs
- Making a diagnosis in a patient with vasculitis is an evolving process because later organ system involvement may result in revision of the initial diagnosis.
- Vasculitis should be considered in patients with constitutional symptoms in conjunction with multisystem disease, palpable purpura, unexplained neurologic symptoms, decreased pulses, bruits, or elevated inflammatory indices.
- Physical findings may be minimal especially early in the course of the disease.

Classification

Large-sized vessel vasculitis	• **Temporal arteritis** - Granulomatous arteritis of the aorta and major branches, especially the extracranial branches of the carotid artery, that usually occurs in patients > 50 years of age • **Takayasu arteritis** - Granulomatous arteritis of the aorta and major branches that usually occurs in patients < 50 years of age
Medium-sized vessel vasculitis	• **Polyarteritis nodosa** - Necrotizing vasculitis of medium-sized or small-sized arteries without involvement of large arteries, veins, or venules; renal involvement without glomerulonephritis • **Kawasaki disease** - Medium-sized and small-sized arteritis of childhood associated with mucocutaneous lymph node syndrome; most commonly affects coronary arteries, although veins and aorta also may be involved

Small-sized vessel vasculitis	• **Wegener granulomatosis** - Granulomatous inflammation of small-sized to medium-sized vessels involving the respiratory tract; necrotizing glomerulonephritis (common)
	• **Churg-Strauss syndrome** - Eosinophil-rich and granulomatous inflammation involving the respiratory tract and necrotizing vasculitis of small-sized to medium-sized vessels; associated with asthma and eosinophilia
	• **Microscopic polyangiitis (MPA)** - Pauci-immune necrotizing vasculitis involving small-sized and medium-sized vessels; necrotizing glomerulonephritis common; pulmonary capillaritis frequent
	• **Henoch-Schönlein purpura** - Small-vessel vasculitis with immunoglobulin A (IgA) immune deposits; involvement of skin, gut, and glomeruli typical; associated with arthritis or arthralgia
	• **Essential cryoglobulinemic vasculitis** - Vasculitis with cryoglobulin immune deposits affecting arterioles and venules; associated with serum cryoglobulins; skin and glomeruli often involved
	• **Cutaneous leukocytoclastic vasculitis** - Isolated cutaneous vasculitis without systemic vasculitis or glomerulonephritis
	• **Possible thrombophlebitis, or superficial venous thrombosis** - Resulting from vasculitic lesions with endothelial activation; in children, more often due to hypercoagulable states or catheter instrumentation

Diagnosis	
History	History should address any medications, recent or recurrent upper respiratory illness, rashes, skin ulcerations, constitutional symptoms, and central and peripheral neurologic symptoms.

Physical Examination	
Henoch-Schönlein purpura	• Palpable purpura
	• Age of onset younger than 20 years
	• Abdominal pain or bowel angina
	• Positive wall granulocytes on biopsy sample of arteriole or venule
Takayasu Arteritis	• Extremity claudication, especially the upper extremities
	• Age younger than 50 years
	• Decreased brachial artery pulses
	• Blood pressure difference greater than 10 mm Hg in the arms
	• Bruit over subclavian artery or aorta
	• Other frequent findings: fever, weight loss, abdominal pain

Polyarteritis nodosa	• Weight loss of more than 4 kg • Livedo reticularis • Myalgias or arthralgias • Mononeuropathy or polyneuropathy • Diastolic blood pressure greater than 90 mm Hg • Elevated BUN or creatinine levels • Positive polymorphonuclear lymphocytes on artery biopsy
Wegener granulomatosis	• Nasal or oral inflammation • Abnormal findings with fixed infiltrates on chest radiography • Microhematuria • Granulomatous inflammation of artery wall biopsy
Churg–Strauss disease	• Asthma • Eosinophilia • Mononeuropathy or polyneuropathy • Migratory or transitory pulmonary infiltrates • Paranasal sinus pain or tenderness • Extravascular eosinophilia
Diagnostic Tests	
Laboratory investigations	• CBC usually reveals normochromic, normocytic anemia of chronic disease; leukocytosis and thrombocytosis reflect inflammation as acute phase reactants. Serum complement is similarly elevated, except in the entity of hypocomplementemic urticarial vasculitis • Elevated sedimentation rate and CRP • BUN, creatinine, and transaminase levels may be elevated depending on organ involvement. Hypoalbuminemia may be present (suggesting chronicity of illness or protein loss). • Cytoplasmic anti-neutrophil cytoplasmic antibodies (c-ANCAs) are associated with Wegener granulomatosis. c-ANCA may be positive in microscopic polyangiitis (MPA); anti-PR3 (a c-ANCA) findings are often negative. • Perinuclear ANCAs (p-ANCAs) are associated with MPA, inflammatory bowel disease, polyarteritis nodosa, and crescentic glomerulonephritis. ELISA for myeloperoxidase is positive. p-ANCAs are also directed against other antigens, including elastase and lactoferrin. In contrast, more than 90% of c-ANCAs are directed against PR3. • Hepatitis is associated with polyarteritis nodosa and cryoglobulinemia; serology may indicate prior or current infection.
Chest radiography	• Used to screen for pulmonary infiltrates or consolidations in Wegener granulomatosis and MPA. Hilar adenopathy suggests pulmonary sarcoidosis

Angiography or magnetic resonance angiography (MRA)	• May reveal long areas of stenosis or aneurysm-formation in the blood vessels.
Biopsy	• Skin biopsy findings may be used to identify vasculitis, but findings are not specific beyond leukocytoclastic vasculitis • Muscle biopsy can be helpful in polyarteritis nodosa • Renal biopsy findings may show focal segmental glomerulonephritis or crescentic lesions
Treatment	
Treatment goals	Decrease acute inflammation of blood vessels and maintain adequate perfusion of vital organs, while limiting the side effects of potentially toxic therapies
Corticosteroids	Are administered in general to control acute symptoms and laboratory evidence of systemic inflammation
Immuno-suppression	For patients with renal or CNS involvement, immunosuppression with cyclophosphamide, azathioprine, methotrexate, or tumor necrosis factor- (TNF-) blockade may be used
Anticoagulation	Anticoagulation is indicated for any patient with a thrombotic episode and an underlying hypercoagulable state
Endovascular or surgical revas-cularization	Indicated in patients with severe stenotic arterial lesions

3.7 Diseases of Large Vessels

3.7.1 Carotid Artery Stenosis

Epidemiology

- In Western countries, stroke is the third most frequent cause of death, behind cardiac disease and cancer, and is the most common condition associated with permanent disability.
- An atherosclerotic stenosis of the internal carotid artery is responsible for 10% to 20% of all ischemic strokes or transient ischemic attacks (TIAs).
- Noninvasive testing with ultrasound can diagnose carotid stenosis.
- Medical management of carotid stenosis includes optimal antiplatelet therapy, lipid lowering therapy and control of blood pressure.
- Large-scale randomized trials have established the benefit of carotid endarterectomy (CEA) over medical management in patients with symptomatic and, to a lesser degree, asymptomatic carotid artery disease.
- Carotid artery stenting (CAS) has been increasingly advocated as less invasive treatment to surgery.
- Carotid artery stenosis is often associated with atherosclerosis elsewhere, i.e. coronary artery and peripheral artery disease.

Diagnosis

History	TIA, stroke	• Symptoms and signs of internal carotid artery stenosis and occlusion reflect ipsilateral ocular and contralateral cerebral hemisphere ischemia • These may be TIAs or permanent deficit, resulting in cerebral infarction (stroke) • Features of ocular ischemia or infarction include partial or complete blindness in one eye (amaurosis fugax) • Hemispheric signs of cerebral infarction from carotid disease include contralateral homonymous hemianopsia, hemiparesis, and hemisensory loss
	Concomitant coronary artery disease	• Angina, dyspnea, othopnea etc. • Patients may give history of exertional chest discomfort.
	Concomitant peripheral artery disease	Intermittent claudication, nonhealing ulcer, rest pain of the extremities

Physical examination	Blood pressure	Measure blood pressure in both arms to rule out stenosis of great vessels or possible aortic dissection.
	Carotid bruit	An important physical sign of carotid stenosis is a carotid bruit heard over the site of the stenosis. However, a carotid bruit is a poor predictor for the presence of an underlying carotid stenosis.
	Peripheral pulses	Clinicians should palpate bilateral brachial, radial, femoral, popliteal, dorsalis pedis, and posterior tibial pulses to assess for concomitant peripheral arterial disease
	Cardiac examination	Palpation, auscultation to assess for ischemic heart disease manifestations such as gallops, murmurs, cardiomegaly etc.
	Neurological evaluation	A complete neurological examination including NIH stroke scale should be performed if appropriate

Diagnostic Tests	
Duplex sonographic examination	• Current first line evaluation for carotid stenosis • A combination of B-mode imaging and pulse Doppler velocity spectrum analysis • Duplex examination is a very reliable, painless, noninvasive, and relatively inexpensive test.
Magnetic resonance (MR) angiography	• Alternative diagnostic test for carotid stenosis • With gadolinium, the test is noninvasive and does not require iodinated contrast • Gadolinium can cause significant skin lesions, particularly in patients with abnormal kidney function, and may cause nephrogenic systemic fibrosis or nephrogenic fibrosing dermopathy.
Computerized tomography (CT) angiography	• Also an alternative diagnostic test for carotid stenosis • Frequently used, often to delineate the extent of the disease including the intracranial component • Contrast angiography is typically indicated for nondiagnostic, noninvasive tests and/or prior to carotid stenting.

Treatment		
Risk factor reduction	Hypertension treatment	• The most important treatable risk factor for stroke-risk reduction • The choice of antihypertensive agent for patients with carotid artery stenosis does not differ from that of hypertensive patients in the general population. • Unless there are indications for specific antihypertensive drugs, patients should be started on a low-dose thiazide diuretic.
	Smoking cessation	Current guidelines recommend smoking cessation for patients with stroke or TIA.
	Cholesterol reduction	• An established risk factor for atherosclerosis • Long-term treatment with statins reduces the risk of stroke • The 2008 American Heart Association / American Stroke Association (AHA/ASA) recommendations state that administration of statin therapy with intensive lipid-lowering effects is recommended for patients with atherosclerotic ischemic stroke or TIA and without known CHD to reduce the risk of stroke and cardiovascular events.
	Antiplatelet therapy	• Almost all patients with TIA or ischemic stroke of atherosclerotic origin also should receive an antiplatelet agent. • The 2008 Update to the AHA/ASA Recommendations for the Prevention of Stroke in Patients With Stroke and Transient Ischemic Attack recommends that aspirin (50 to 325 mg/d) monotherapy, the combination of aspirin and extended-release dipyridamole, and clopidogrel monotherapy all are acceptable options for initial antiplatelet therapy.
Carotid endarterectomy (CEA)		• Beneficial for patients with asymptomatic carotid stenosis of 60% to 99 %. However, the number needed to treat to prevent one stroke at three years is ~33, and the degree of benefit is lower compared with symptomatic carotid stenosis. • Recommended for patients with recently symptomatic carotid stenosis of 70% to 99 % who have a life expectancy of at least five years, provided that the perioperative risk of stroke and death for the surgeon or center is < 6%. • Reasonable for men with recently symptomatic carotid stenosis of 50% to 69 % who have a life expectancy of at least five years, provided that the perioperative risk of stroke and death for the surgeon or center is less than 6 percent. • All patients undergoing CEA should receive concomitant secondary preventative therapies including antiplatelet and lipid lowering therapy.

Carotid stenting (CAS)	• The role of carotid artery stenting (CAS) in the treatment of carotid stenosis is not yet well defined. • For patients with recently symptomatic carotid stenosis of 70% to 99% who have a stenosis that is difficult to access surgically, or have severe medical, cardiac, or pulmonary disease that greatly increases the risk of surgery, or radiation-induced stenosis, or restenosis after endarterectomy, CAS is a reasonable option. • CAS should be performed using an emboli-protection device. • Ongoing trials will help further define the role of CAS in low-risk patients.

3.7.2 Renal Artery Stenosis

Epidemiology

Renal artery stenosis or renovascular disease is an important correctable cause of secondary hypertension.

Clinical Features Suggestive of the Presence of Renal Artery Stenosis

• Young or middle-aged female with severe hypertension and no family history (fibromuscular dysplasia)
• Uncontrolled hypertension despite at least three anti-hypertensive agents in adequate doses (regimen includes a diuretic)
• Worsening blood pressure control in compliant, long-standing hypertensive patient
• Acute renal failure or elevation of creatinine with angiotensin converting enzyme inhibitors or angiotensin-receptor blockers
• Chronic renal insufficiency with mild proteinuria and bland urinary sediment
• Recurrent flash pulmonary edema
• > 1.5 cm difference in kidney sizes
• Hypertension with hypokalemia and hyponatremia (secondary hyperaldosteronism due to elevated renin)
• Bruit over the abdominal aorta (lateralizing bruit over the renal arteries is more specific but uncommon)
• Hypertension and concomitant peripheral arterial disease
• Severe hypertensive retinopathy

Diagnosis		
History	Hypertension (uncontrolled, difficult to treat)	• Onset of hypertension before the age of 30 years, particularly if there is a negative family history and no other risk factors for hypertension • Onset of severe or stage II hypertension (blood pressure ≥160/100 mm Hg) in someone > 55 years old and refractory or resistant hypertension, adhering to therapeutic doses of three appropriate antihypertensive agents (including a diuretic), should alert the clinician to the presence of secondary hypertension which may be due to renal artery stenosis
Physical Examination	Blood pressure	Measure blood pressure in both arms and the leg to rule out coarctation.
	Abdominal bruit	Occasionally, a bruit may be heart over a stenotic renal artery in a relatively thin patient.
	Peripheral pulses	Clinicians should palpate bilateral brachial, radial, femoral, popliteal, dorsalis pedis, and posterior tibial pulses to assess for concomitant peripheral arterial disease. Atherosclerotic renal artery stenosis may accompany PAD.
	Cardiac Examination	Palpation, auscultation to assess for hypertensive heart disease manifestations such as gallops, murmurs, cardiomegaly etc.

Diagnostic Tests	
• The American College of Cardiology/American Heart Association (ACC/AHA) guidelines on Peripheral Arterial Disease state that screening for renal artery stenosis only is indicated if revascularization would be considered if clinically significant renovascular disease was detected • The choice of test should be based upon institutional expertise and pertinent patient factors	
MR angiography	• Increasingly used as the first-line screening test for renovascular hypertension • Among patients with moderate to severe renal disease, the administration of gadolinium has been linked to a severe disease called nephrogenic systemic fibrosis. • It is recommended that gadolinium-based imaging should not be used in patients with an estimated glomerular filtration rate less than 30 mL/min.
CTA	Another highly accurate noninvasive screening test of choice in screening for renovascular hypertension

Duplex Doppler sonography	• May detect both unilateral and bilateral disease in appropriate patients. • This modality also can be used to detect recurrent stenosis in patients previously treated with stenting or surgery.
Catheter angiography	Recommended if the noninvasive tests are inconclusive or nondiagnostic, and the clinical suspicion is high

Captopril renal scintigraphy, selective renal vein renin measurements, and plasma renin activity are no longer recommended as screening tests for renal artery stenosis

Treatment	
The optimal treatment of renal artery stenosis depends upon a number of factors including the etiology of the stenosis, the location of the stenosis, and patient preference	
Pharmacological treatment	• ACE inhibitors, ARBs and calcium-channel blockers are effective medications for treatment of hypertension associated with unilateral RAS. • Patients with bilateral RAS who are not good revascularization candidates or refuse an invasive procedure can be treated with medical therapy (beginning with an ACE inhibitor or ARB and, if necessary, a diuretic) as long as the BP can be adequately controlled and renal function is reasonably maintained. • A calcium channel blocker can be added or substituted if there is a significant drug-induced rise in the serum creatinine concentration, because calcium channel blockers are more likely to dilate the afferent arteriole and therefore maintain the GFR
Revascularization	• May be indicated in patients with a hemodynamically significant lesion who have resistant hypertension, malignant hypertension, hypertension with an otherwise unexplained unilateral small kidney, an inability to tolerate antihypertensive medications, recurrent episodes of flash pulmonary edema, and unstable angina or acute coronary syndrome • The procedure of choice in most centers at the present time is percutaneous angioplasty with stent implantation.
Percutaneous revascularization	• Indicated for patients with hemodynamically significant renal artery stenosis and recurrent, unexplained congestive heart failure or sudden, unexplained pulmonary edema • Also reasonable for patients with RAS and progressive chronic kidney disease with bilateral RAS or RAS due to a solitary functioning kidney
Surgical revascularization	Performed if angioplasty fails or in those who require aortic reconstruction near the renal arteries for other indications such as aneurysm or dissection repair

3.7.3   Aortic Dissection and aneurysm

Epidemiology

- Acute aortic dissection is a medical emergency with high morbidity and mortality requiring emergent diagnosis and therapy.
- Data concerning the incidence of acute aortic dissection in the general population are limited and estimates range from 2.6-3.5 per 100 000 person-years
- The most important predisposing factor for acute aortic dissection is systemic hypertension.
- The primary event in aortic dissection is a tear in the aortic intima. Degeneration of the aortic media, or cystic medial necrosis, is felt to be necessary for the development of aortic dissection.
- An aneurysm is currently defined as a localized dilatation of the aorta, 50% over the normal diameter, which includes all three layers of the vessel (intima, media, and adventitia).
- The incidence of thoracic aortic aneurysm is estimated to be 6-10 cases per 100,000 patient-years.
- The prevalence of abdominal aortic aneurysms is negligible in individuals under the age of 60 y and then increases dramatically with age, occuring in 4% to 9% of individuals > 60 years of age.

Types of Aortic Dissection

- Classification of aortic dissection is based upon the site of the intimal tear and the extent of the dissecting hematoma.
- Two different classification systems, the DeBakey and Stanford systems, have been used to classify aortic dissection, with the Stanford system being more popular and clinically used

DeBakey	Type I	• The intimal tear is located in the ascending aorta, usually just a few centimeters above the aortic valve. • The hematoma extends for a variable distance beyond the ascending aorta.
	Type II	• The intimal tear is located in the ascending aorta, usually just a few centimeters above the aortic valve. • The dissecting hematoma is confined to the ascending aorta.
	Type III	• The dissection originates in the descending aorta, typically just beyond the origin of the left subclavian artery and propagates antegrade into the descending aorta or, rarely, retrograde into the aortic arch and ascending aorta.
Stanford	Type A	• Refers to all dissections that involve the ascending aorta, and the entry site may be located anywhere along the course of the aorta.
	Type B	• All other dissections are classified as type B. • In type B, the dissection is confined to the aorta distal to the left subclavian artery.

Diagnosis		
History	Chest pain	• Typical features of dissection are the acute/ instantaneous onset of chest and/or back pain of sharp, severe, and sometimes radiating and migrating nature.
	Predisposing fact.	• A history of, or signs of chronic hypertension usually are seen if obvious signs of connective tissue disorders are absent.
	Syncope	• Up to 20% of patients with acute aortic dissection may present with syncope, without a history of typical pain or neurological findings. • Cardiac tamponade may result in hypotension and syncope. • Syncope also may result from severe pain, obstruction of cerebral vessels, or activation of aortic baroreceptors.
	Dyspnea	• After an initial presentation of chest pain, heart failure may become the main symptom and usually is related to severe aortic regurgitation.
	Abdominal pain	• Recurrent abdominal pain, elevation of acute phase reactants, and increase of lactate dehydrogenase (LDH) indicate involvement of either the celiac trunk (in approximately 8%) or the mesenteric artery (in approximately 8% to 13%).
	Oliguria/ anuria	• Involvement of the renal arteries may result in oliguria, anuria, or acute renal failure.
Physical examination	Pulse deficit	• Pulse deficits on physical examination are important but uncommon clues to the presence of aortic dissection. • In the International Registry of Aortic Dissection (IRAD), pulse deficits were reported in < 20% of patients.
	Cardiac murmur	• A diastolic murmur indicative of aortic regurgitation is seen in 40% to 50% of patients with proximal dissection.
	Elevated JVP	• Signs of pericardial involvement, jugular venous distension, or a paradoxical pulse should alert the physician to a rapidly worsening clinical scenario.
	Blood pressure	• Shock may be a presenting sign, resulting from tamponade, coronary compression, acute aortic valve incompetence, or loss of blood and imminent exsanguinations • Blood pressure may be unequal in both arms if great vessels are involved.
	Neurological evaluation	• A complete neurological exam including a NIH stroke scale should be performed if there is evidence of stroke.

Diagnostic Tests

- Rapid diagnosis of aortic dissection is imperative due to the potentially catastrophic nature of the illness and the exceedingly high mortality if not diagnosed early in the course.
- Mediastinal and/or aortic widening on chest radiograph may be evident and may suggest dissection.
- Various imaging modalities are available for the definitive diagnosis of aortic dissection including transthoracic echocardiography (TTE), transesophageal echocardiography (TEE), computed tomography (CT), magnetic resonance imaging (MRI), and contrast aortography.

CT scan	Advantages include ready availability at most hospitals, even on an emergency basis, and identification of thrombus and pericardial effusion
MRI	A highly accurate noninvasive technique for evaluating the aorta in patients with suspected dissection, but is less readily available and has other logistical disadvantages such as the requirement for patients to remain motionless with relatively limited access for > 30 minutes
TEE	• TTE has limited utility for evaluation of the aorta for dissection • Multiplane TEE on the other hand has very high sensitivity and specificity and can be performed bedside
Aortography	Has generally been replaced in the current era by noninvasive testing to establish the diagnosis of aortic dissection

All of the diagnostic modalities discussed above also may be used to identify aortic aneurysms.

Acute Treatment

- Patients with suspected aortic dissection should be admitted to an intensive care unit as rapidly as possible after confirmation of the diagnosis, and reduction of systolic blood pressure to 100–120 mm Hg should be attempted
- For blood pressure control, initial treatment consists of an intravenous β-Blocker to reduce the heart rate below 60 beats/min; the associated fall in both blood pressure and the rate of rise in systolic pressure will minimize aortic wall stress. Labetalol or esmolol are the preferred agents. Verapamil or diltiazem may be used in patients who cannot tolerate β-Blockers.
- Sodium nitroprusside should be used if systolic blood pressure remains > 100 mm Hg despite adequate β-Blockade.
- Acute dissections involving the ascending aorta are considered surgical emergencies
- Dissections confined to the descending aorta are treated medically unless the patient demonstrates progression or complications.
- Stenting and/or balloon fenestration of the dissecting membrane may be considered for patients with a type A dissection in whom mesenteric, renal, or peripheral ischemia persists after surgical repair or for patients with a type B dissection treated medically in whom mesenteric, renal, or peripheral ischemic complications develop.

Long-term Treatment		
β-Blocker therapy	Treatment with effective β-Blockade is an important component of long term medical therapy.	
Calcium antagonists	Although limited data exist for their use for the long-term management of aortic dissection, these agents remain a reasonable alternative for those patients who are intolerant of β-Blockers.	
Blood pressure and fasting serum lipid values	Should be monitored and controlled as recommended for patients with atherosclerotic disease	
Follow-up imaging and examination	Recommendations are for follow-up imaging for every patient with aortic dissection and examination at 1, 3, 6, 9, and 12 months after discharge and annually thereafter.	
Infrarenal or juxta-renal AAAs measuring 5.5 cm or larger	Should undergo repair to eliminate the risk of rupture	
Infrarenal or juxta-renal AAAs measuring 4.0–5.4 cm in diameter	Should be monitored by ultrasound or computed tomography (CT) scans every 6 to 12 months to detect expansion	
Thoracic aortic aneurysm with size between 5–6 cm	Elective surgery	
	Open repair	Open repair of infrarenal AAAs and/or common iliac aneurysms is indicated in patients who are good or average surgical candidates.
	Endovascular repair	Endovascular repair of infrarenal aortic and/or common iliac aneurysms is reasonable in patients at high risk of complications from open operations because of cardiopulmonary or other associated diseases.
AAA = abdominal aortic aneurysm		

3.7.4 Peripheral Arterial Disease

Epidemiology

- Peripheral arterial disease (PAD) refers to stenotic, occlusive, and aneurysmal diseases of the aorta and its branch arteries, exclusive of the coronary arteries.
- The prevalence of PAD increases progressively with age, beginning after age 40 y
- Risk factors for PAD include diabetes, smoking, dyslipidemia, and hypertension
- In the 1999 to 2000 National Health and Nutrition Examination Survey (NHANES) survey, the prevalence of PAD was 0.9 % between the ages of 40 and 49 y, 2.5% between the ages of 50 and 59 y, 4.7% between the ages of 60 and 69 y, and 14.5% age 70 y and older.

Individuals at Risk for PAD

- Age < 50 years, with diabetes and one other atherosclerosis risk factor (smoking, dyslipidemia, hypertension, or hyperhomocysteinemia)
- Age 50 to 69 years and history of smoking or diabetes
- Age 70 years and older
- Leg symptoms with exertion (suggestive of claudication) or ischemic rest pain
- Abnormal lower extremity pulse examination
- Known atherosclerotic coronary, carotid, or renal artery disease

Diagnosis

Patients with PAD often present with symptoms of leg ischemia. However, up to 50% of patients are asymptomatic, and, among symptomatic patients, atypical symptoms are more common than classic intermittent claudication.

History	Intermittent claudication	Exertional limitation of the lower extremity muscles or any history of walking impairment (described as fatigue, aching, numbness, or pain in the buttock, thigh, calf, or foot). The relationship between the site of pain and level of arterial disease is summarized below: • Buttock and hip - aortoiliac disease • Thigh - common femoral artery or aortoiliac disease • Upper two-thirds of the calf - superficial femoral artery • Lower one-third of the calf - popliteal artery • Foot claudication - tibial or peroneal artery
	Nonhealing ulcer	• Any poorly healing or nonhealing wounds of the legs or feet
	Rest pain	• Any pain at rest localized to the lower leg or foot and its association with the upright or recumbent positions
	Family history	• Family history of a first-degree relative with an abdominal aortic aneurysm (AAA)

Physical examination	Pulses	• Palpation of pulses at the brachial, radial, ulnar, femoral, popliteal, dorsalis pedis, and posterior tibial sites • Perform Allen's test when knowledge of hand perfusion is needed • Pulse intensity assessed and should be recorded numerically as follows: 0, absent; 1, diminished; 2, normal; 3, bounding
	Blood Pressure	• Measure of blood pressure in both arms and document any in-terarm differences
	Feet	• The shoes and socks should be removed; the feet inspected; the color, temperature, and integrity of the skin and intertriginous areas evaluated; and the presence of ulcerations recorded.
	Local changes	• Additional findings suggestive of severe PAD, including distal hair loss, trophic skin changes, and hypertrophic nails, should be sought and recorded.

Diagnostic Tests	
Laboratory	• The noninvasive vascular laboratory provides a powerful set of tools that can objectively assess the status of lower extremity arterial disease and facilitate the creation of a therapeutic plan.

Ankle–brachial index (ABI)	• A relatively simple method to confirm the clinical suspicion of PAD
	• Provides a measure of the severity of PAD
	• Calculation of the ABI is performed by measuring the systolic blood pressure (by Doppler probe) in the brachial, posterior tibial, and dorsalis pedis arteries.
	• The highest of the measurements in the ankles of feet is divided by the higher of the two brachial measurements
	  - The normal ABI is 1.0 - 1.3, since the pressure is higher in the ankle than in the arm. Values > 1.30 are abnormal and suggest a noncompressible calcified vessel.
	  - An ABI < 0.9 has 95% sensitivity (and 100% specificity) for detecting angiogram-positive PAD and is associated with ≥ 50% stenosis in one or more major vessels.
	  - An ABI of 0.40 to 0.90 suggests a degree of arterial obstruction often associated with claudication.
	  - An ABI < 0.4 represents severe ischemia.
	• Post-exercise ABI may be helpful in identifying patients with moderate stenosis.

Segmental limb pressures	• For assessment of the level and extent of PAD • A 20 mm Hg or greater reduction in pressure is considered significant if such a gradient is present either between segments along the same leg or when compared to the same level in the opposite leg.
Plethysmography and pulse volume recorders	• Plethysmography, or the measurement of volume change in an organ or limb, is usually used in conjunction with segmental limb pressures to assess the level of arterial disease. • This technique is performed by injecting a standard volume of air into pneumatic cuffs placed at various levels along the extremity. • Volume changes in the limb segment below the cuff are translated into pulsatile pressure, which is detected by a transducer and then displayed as a pressure-pulse contour. • Pulse volume recordings (PVR) are most useful in detecting disease in calcified vessels which tend to yield falsely elevated pressures. **(NOTE: Do not do segmental pressures and PVRs in patient with known or suspected acute DVT).**
Duplex sonography	• Lower extremity arteries can be examined. • Assessment begins at the common femoral artery and proceeds distally to the popliteal artery. • An area of stenosis is localized with color Doppler and assessed by measuring Doppler velocities at several arterial sites.
CTA	• A useful modality for the detection of aortic and lower extremity PAD. • The sensitivity and specificity for detecting a stenosis of at least 50% are 95% and 96%, respectively, compared with traditional digital subtraction angiography.
MR angiography	Another noninvasive modality that is helpful to assess extent and severity of PAD
Contrast angiography	Remains the gold standard but is primarily used prior to revascularization

Treatment	
Risk factor reduction	• Smoking cessation, lipid lowering, and diabetes and hypertension treatment according to current national treatment guidelines are recommended for individuals with asymptomatic lower extremity PAD • Cessation of cigarette smoking reduces the progression of disease as shown by lower amputation rates and lower incidences of rest ischemia among those who quit completely. • Antiplatelet therapy is indicated for individuals with asymptomatic lower extremity PAD to reduce the risk of adverse cardiovascular ischemic events.
Exercise rehabilitation programs	• Several studies have demonstrated the benefit of exercise rehabilitation programs in reducing symptoms of claudication. • Exercise rehabilitation programs consist of a series of sessions lasting 45 to 60 minutes per session, involving use of either a treadmill or a track to permit each patient to achieve symptom-limited claudication. • The initial session usually includes 35 minutes of intermittent walking; walking is then increased by five minutes each session until 50 minutes of intermittent walking can be accomplished. Warm-up and cool down sessions of five to ten minutes each are included. • The patient should attend at least three sessions per week, with a program length > 3 months.
Pharmacological therapy	• **Cilostazol** (100 mg orally 2 times per day) is indicated as an effective therapy to improve symptoms and increase walking distance in patients with lower extremity PAD and intermittent claudication (in the absence of HF). • A therapeutic trial of cilostazol is reasonable in all patients with lifestyle-limiting claudication (in the absence of HF). • **Pentoxifylline** (400 mg 3 times per day) may be considered as second-line alternative therapy to cilostazol to improve walking distance in patients with intermittent claudication. • It should be noted that the clinical effectiveness of pentoxifylline as therapy for claudication is marginal and not well established. • **Chelation** (e.g., ethylenediaminetetraacetic acid) **is not indicated** for treatment of intermittent claudication and may have harmful adverse effects.

Revascularization procedures (surgical or endovascular)	• Patients with intermittent claudication should have significant functional impairment, with a reasonable likelihood of symptomatic improvement, and absence of other disease that would comparably limit exercise even if the claudication was improved (e.g., angina, heart failure, chronic respiratory disease, or orthopedic limitations) before undergoing consideration for revascularization • Indicated for individuals with a lifestyle-limiting disability due to intermittent claudication when clinical features suggest a reasonable likelihood of symptomatic improvement with endovascular intervention and (a) there has been an inadequate response to exercise or pharmacological therapy and/or (b) there is a very favorable risk-benefit ratio (e.g., focal aorto-iliac occlusive disease) (see following Figure) • Catheter-based thrombolysis is an effective and beneficial therapy and is indicated for patients with acute limb ischemia present for less than 14 days.

Summary of Preferred Options in Interventional Management of Iliac Lesions

Type A Endovascular Treatment of Choice	Type B Currently, endovascular treatment is more often used but insufficient evidence for recommendation	Type C Currently, surgical treatment is more often used but insufficient evidence for recommendation	Type D Surgical treatment of choice

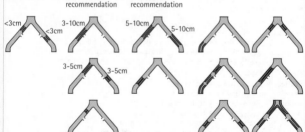

Reprinted from Journal of Vascular Surgery, 31 (1, part 2), Dormandy JA et al., Endovascular procedures for intermittent claudication, S97–S113, Copyright 2000, with permission from Elsevier.

3.8   Cardiomyopathies

3.8.1   Dilated Cardiomyopathy (DCM)

Epidemiology

- Refers to the subset of cardiomyopathies characterized by dilation and contractile dysfunction of the left and right ventricles
- A common and largely irreversible form of heart muscle disease with an estimated prevalence of 1:2500 people
- The third most common cause of heart failure and the most frequent cause of heart transplantation

Causes

- Alcohol (chronic heavy consumption)
- Other drugs (heavy metals, anthracyclines [daunorubicin and doxorubicin], cocaine, methamphetamine, cobalt)
- Infections (viral endocarditis/myocarditis [coxsackievirus, adenovirus, parvovirus, human immunodeficiency virus, HIV], Chagas disease [most common cause in parts of South America])
- High-output states (anemia, thyrotoxicosis, pregnancy)
- Collagen vascular disease
- Glycogen storage disease (type IV also known as Andersen disease is associated with DCM)
- Thiamine deficiency and zinc deficiency
- Hypophosphatemia
- Amyloidosis
- Neuromuscular disorders (Duchenne or Becker and Emery-Dreifuss muscular dystrophies)
- Pheochromocytoma

Diagnosis

History	Symptoms (good indicator of the severity of the disease)	• Fatigue • Dyspnea on exertion, shortness of breath • Orthopnea, paroxysmal nocturnal dyspnea • Increasing edema, weight, or abdominal girth
Physical examination	Signs of heart failure and volume overload	• Tachypnea • Tachycardia • Hypertension • Hypoxia • Jugular venous distension (JVD) • Pulmonary edema (crackles and/or wheezes) • S_3 gallop • Enlarged liver or presence of hepatojugular reflex • Peripheral edema

Diagnostic Tests	
Laboratory testing	Elevated plasma brain natriuretic peptide (BNP) is useful in diagnosing heart failure
Chest radiography	Pulmonary vascular congestion may be observed
ECG	Often shows non-specific ST-T wave changes, intraventricular conduction delay, and bundle branch block pattern
Echocardiography	• Plays a pivotal role in the diagnosis and classification of cardiomyopathy • Allows assessment of systolic and diastolic function
Magnetic resonance (MR) imaging	MRI with gadolinium has been used to evaluate the extent of mid-wall fibrosis, which may correlate with risk of arrhythmias and failure to respond to treatment
Right-sided heart catheterization (RHC)	Can be beneficial in determining the volume status of a patient with equivocal clinical signs and symptoms of heart failure and assessing pulmonary vascular resistance

Treatment		
Pharmaco-therapy	General information	• The goals of pharmacotherapy are to treat symptoms of heart failure. • Long-term treatment follows the same medical regimen, including ACE inhibitors, beta blockers, diuretics and aldosterone receptor antagonists.
	ACE inhibitors and β-Blockers	• Constitute current standard in the treatment of left ventricular dysfunction
	Diuretics	• May be needed to treat pulmonary and systemic congestion
	Aldosterone antagonists	• Are complementary to standard therapy in modulating the RAAS because aldosterone levels remain elevated despite ACE inhibitor therapy
	Inotropic drugs	• e.g. dobutamine, milrinone • May be necessary for severe decompensation
Invasive therapy	Ventricular assist devices and cardiac transplantation	Options for severe refractory heart failure

3.8.2 Hypertrophic Cardiomyopathy (HCM)

Epidemiology

- A primary cardiac disorder that results from known or suspected genetic defects in sarcomeric proteins of the cardiac myocyte
- The condition is characterized by myocardial hypertrophy that is inappropriate, asymmetric, and occurs in the absence of an obvious inciting hypertrophy stimulus.
- Although any region of the left ventricle (LV) may be affected, hypertrophy frequently involves the interventricular septum, which can result in outflow tract obstruction.
- Patients typically have preserved or hyperdynamic systolic function with impaired LV compliance that results in diastolic dysfunction, whether or not outflow tract obstruction is present.
- HCM is reported in 0.5% of the outpatient population referred for echocardiography.

Pathophysiology

- There is evidence of dynamic pressure gradient across the LV outflow tract.
- The pressure gradient appears to be related to asymmetric septal hypertrophy and abnormal systolic anterior motion of the mitral valve against the hypertrophied septum.
- In addition, most patients have abnormal diastolic function.

Diagnosis

History	Sudden cardiac death	• Sudden cardiac death is the most devastating presenting manifestation of HCM .
	Dyspnea	• The most common presenting symptom, occurring in as many as 90% of symptomatic patients.
	Syncope	• A fairly common symptom, resulting from inadequate cardiac output upon exertion or from cardiac arrhythmia
	Angina	• Typical symptoms of angina are quite common in patients with HCM and may occur in the absence of detectable coronary atherosclerosis
	Palpitations	• Palpitations are common and result from arrhythmias, such as premature atrial and ventricular beats, sinus pauses, atrial fibrillation, atrial flutter, supraventricular tachycardia, and ventricular tachycardia.

Physical examination	Double apical impulse	• Results from a forceful left atrial contraction against a highly noncompliant left ventricle and seen quite commonly in adults
	Triple apical impulse	• Results from a late systolic bulge that occurs when the heart is almost empty and is performing near-isometric contraction. • This is a highly characteristic finding of HCM but seen less frequently than the double apical impulse
	Fourth heart sound	• S_4 is frequently heard and results from atrial systole against a highly noncompliant stiff left ventricle.
	Systolic ejection murmur	• Best heard between the apex and left sternal border; radiates to the suprasternal notch but not to the carotid arteries or neck. • The murmur and the gradient across the LV outflow tract diminish with any increase in preload (e.g., Mueller maneuver, squatting) or increase in afterload (e.g., handgrip). • The murmur and the gradient increase with any decrease in preload (e.g., Valsalva maneuver, nitrate administration, diuretic administration, standing) or with any decrease in afterload (e.g., vasodilator administration).

Diagnostic Tests	
ECG	• Often shows evidence of left ventricular hypertrophy. • Other findings observed on ECG include axis deviation (usually left), conduction abnormalities (PR prolongation, bundle-branch block), sinus bradycardia with ectopic atrial rhythm, and atrial enlargement.
Echocardiography	• Doppler studies in patients with obstructive HCM reveal an elevated flow velocity across the LV outflow tract • Diastolic dysfunction with reduced LV compliance and a mitral valve ratio of E wave to A wave of less than 1 (usually < 0.8) • Systolic anterior motion of the anterior mitral valve leaflet and asymmetric septal hypertrophy with a ratio of septal wall thickness to posterior wall thickness of greater than 1.4:1 • A summary of echocardiographic findings includes abnormal systolic anterior leaflet motion of the mitral valve, LV hypertrophy, left atrial enlargement, small ventricular chamber size, septal hypertrophy with septal-to-free wall ratio greater than 1.4:1, mitral valve prolapse and mitral regurgitation, decreased mid aortic flow, and partial systolic closure of the aortic valve in mid systole.

Magnetic resonance (MR) imaging		• MRI with gadolinium has been used to evaluate HCM and may reveal scar tissue.
Cardiac catheterization		• Useful to determine the degree of outflow obstruction, cardiac hemodynamics, diastolic characteristics of the left ventricle and LV anatomy, and, of particular importance, the coronary anatomy.
Postextrasystolic potentiation		• A potent stimulus for enhancing the left ventricular outflow gradient is postextrasystolic potentiation, which may occur after a spontaneous premature contraction or be induced by mechanical stimulation with a catheter. • The resultant increase in contractility in the beat after the extrasystole produces an increase in the outflow gradient. • A characteristic change often occurs in the directly recorded arterial pressure tracing, which, in addition to displacing a more marked spike and dome configuration, exhibits a pulse pressure that fails to increase as expected or actually decreases (the Brockenbrough-Braunwald phenomenon).

Treatment			
Pharmaco-therapy	General information		• The purpose of pharmacologic therapy is to reduce the pressure gradient across the LV outflow tract by reducing the inotropic state of the left ventricle, improving compliance of the left ventricle, and reducing diastolic dysfunction.
	β-Blockers		• Reduce inotropic state of left ventricle, improve diastolic function, and increase LV compliance, thereby reducing pressure gradient across LV outflow tract
	Disopyramide		• Decreases inotropic state of left ventricle, decreases ventricular and supraventricular arrhythmias, decreases diastolic dysfunction and increases LV compliance, reducing the pressure gradient across the LV outflow tract
	Calcium channel blockers		• An alternative to β-Blockers • Decrease inotropic state of the left ventricle, decrease gradient across the LV outflow tract, decrease diastolic dysfunction, and increase diastolic filling of the left ventricle by improving LV diastolic relaxation

Invasive therapy	LV myomectomy	• Used for patients with severe symptoms refractory to therapy and an outflow gradient of more than 50 mm Hg, either with provocation or with rest
	Transcatheter septal alcohol ablation	• Also may be used to relieve the LV outflow obstruction caused by infarction of a portion of the interventricular septum
	Implantable cardioverter defibrillators (ICD)	• Have been used for the prevention of sudden arrhythmic death

3.8.3 Restrictive Cardiomyopathy (RCM)

Epidemiology

- The least common form of cardiomyopathy
- The condition is characterized by restrictive filling and reduced diastolic volume of either or both ventricles with normal or near-normal systolic function and wall thickness.
- This disease may be idiopathic or associated with other diseases (e.g., amyloidosis, hemochromatosis, endomyocardial disease with or without hypereosinophilia).
- **It is critical to distinguish RCM from constrictive pericarditis, which also presents with restrictive physiology but is frequently curable by surgical intervention**

Pathophysiology

- There is increased stiffness of the myocardium, which causes pressure within the ventricles to rise precipitously with small increases in volume.
- The pressure gradient appears to be related to asymmetric septal hypertrophy and abnormal systolic anterior motion of the mitral valve against the hypertrophied septum.
- In addition, most patients have abnormal diastolic function.

Causes

- Idiopathic
- Infiltrative
  - Amyloidosis
  - Hemochromatosis (dilated left ventricle with restrictive physiology)
  - Glycogen-storage disease
  - Treatment-induced(following heart transplantation, following mediastinal radiation)
  - Malignancy (metastatic endocardial and myocardial infiltration, carcinoid heart disease)
- Eosinophilic cardiomyopathy and endomyocardial fibrosis
- Postirradiation fibrosis
  - The differential between constriction and restriction may be particularly difficult in these patients because the 2 conditions may coexist.

Diagnosis		
History	Dyspnea	• Patients usually complain of gradually worsening shortness of breath, progressive exercise intolerance, and fatigue.
	Fatigue	• Fatigue and weakness are results of decreased stroke volume and cardiac output.
	Ascites, edema	• Patients may have distention of the abdomen secondary to ascites, and they frequently have profound bilateral peripheral edema.
	Angina	• Chest pain secondary to angina or chest pain mimicking myocardial ischemia can be observed, primarily in patients with amyloidosis, possibly due to myocardial compression of small vessels
	Palpitations	• Patients may complain of palpitations, frequently due to atrial fibrillation, which is common in RCM.
	Thrombo-embolic complications	• As many as a third of patients with idiopathic RCM may present with thromboembolic complications, especially pulmonary emboli secondary to DVT.
	General	• Depending on the etiology, patients may have a prior history of radiation therapy, heart transplantation, chemotherapy, or a systemic disease.
Physical examination	Signs of amyloidosis	• Easy bruising, periorbital purpura, macroglossia, and other systemic findings, such as carpal tunnel syndrome, should advise the clinician to consider amyloidosis.
	Increased jugular venous pressure	• Increased jugular venous pressure is present, with rapid x and y descents. • The most prominent finding is usually the rapid y descent. • The degree of elevation of the jugular venous pressure indicates the severity of impaired filling of the right ventricle.
	Loud early diastolic filling sound (S_3)	• A loud early diastolic filling sound (S_3) may be present but is uncommon in amyloidosis.
	Ascites, Edema	• Patients frequently have ascites and pitting edema of the lower extremities

Diagnostic Tests	
Laboratory testing	• Complete blood count with peripheral smear may show eosinophilia in eosinophilic cardiomyopathy.
	• Serum iron concentrations, percent saturation of total iron-binding capacity, and serum ferritin levels all are increased in hemochromatosis.
	• Serum BNP levels are nearly normal or mildly elevated in patients with constrictive physiology of heart failure, and grossly elevated in patients with restrictive physiology, despite nearly identical clinical and hemodynamic presentation
Chest radiography	• Typically shows cardiomegaly with bilateral pleural effusions
Echocardiography	• Shows a nondilated, normally contracting, nonhypertrophied left ventricle and marked dilatation of both atria
	• Granular speckling of the ventricular walls suggests the presence of infiltrative disease, such as amyloidosis.
	• Doppler echocardiogram shows accentuated early diastolic filling of the ventricles (E), shortened deceleration time, and diminished atrial filling (A), which results in a high E-to-A ratio on the mitral inflow velocities.
	• Respiratory variations of diastolic (transmitral) blood flow help to differentiate between constrictive pericarditis and restrictive cardiomyopathy (RCM).
	• A pattern of respiratory variation, with a diminished peak transmitral diastolic flow during inspiration, is characteristic of pericardial constriction but not of RCM.
Magnetic resonance (MR) imaging	• May show a characteristic pattern of global subendocardial late gadolinium enhancement in RCM
Cardiac catheterization	• Shows increased right heart pressures and the dip-plateau or square-root contour of the ventricular diastolic pressures (deep and rapid early decline in ventricular pressure at the onset of diastole, with a rapid rise to a plateau in early diastole)

Treatment		
General measures	General information	• The purpose of therapy is to reduce symptoms by lowering elevated filling pressures without significantly reducing the cardiac output.
	Diuretics	• Current therapy consists predominantly of low-dose diuretics to lower the preload.
	Caution with ACE inhibitors and angiotensin II inhibitors	• Are poorly tolerated in patients with amyloidosis and even small doses may result in profound hypotension, probably secondary to an autonomic neuropathy
	Anticoagulation	• Patients with a history of embolization or atrial fibrillation should be anticoagulated.
	Cardiac transplantation	• Can be considered in highly selected patients with refractory symptoms in idiopathic or familial RCM and amyloidosis
Disease-specific measures	Antiplasma cell therapy	• With melphalan • May slow the progress of systemic amyloidosis by stopping production of the paraprotein responsible for the formation of amyloid
	Corticosteroids, cytotoxic agents, interferon	• Medical therapy with corticosteroids, cytotoxic agents (e.g., hydroxyurea), and interferon is appropriate during the early phase of Loeffler endocarditis and improves symptoms and survival.
	Chelation therapy or phlebotomy	• Effective in patients with hemochromatosis to decrease the iron overload

3.8.4 Constrictive Pericarditis

Epidemiology

- Constrictive pericarditis is characterized by a thickened fibrotic pericardium, which impedes normal diastolic filling.
- The classic diagnostic conundrum of constrictive pericarditis is the difficulty in distinguishing it from restrictive cardiomyopathy (RCM).
- The frequency of a diagnosis of constrictive pericarditis is less than 1 in 10 000 hospital admissions.

Pathophysiology

- Since the myocardium is unaffected, early ventricular filling during the first third of diastole is unimpeded, but afterwards, the stiff pericardium affects flow and hemodynamics.
- The ventricular pressure decreases rapidly early (producing a steep y descent on right atrial pressure waveform tracings) and then increases abruptly to a level that is sustained until systole.
- Clinical symptoms are related to early rapid diastolic filling, and elevation and equalization of the diastolic pressures in all of the cardiac chambers restricting late diastolic filling, leading to venous engorgement and decreased cardiac output, all secondary to a confining pericardium.

Causes

- Idiopathic
- Infectious (bacterial): Tuberculosis is the leading cause of constrictive pericarditis in developing nations but represents only a minority of causes in the United States and other developed countries.
- Infectious (viral): Coxsackie virus, hepatitis, adenovirus, and echovirus.
- Radiation-induced
- Postsurgical: Any operative or invasive (catheterization) procedure in which the pericardium is opened, manipulated, or damaged may invoke an inflammatory response, leading to constrictive pericarditis.
- Uremia: Constrictive pericarditis may develop in association with long-term hemodialysis.
- Drug-induced: Procainamide and hydralazine have been reported to cause constrictive pericarditis through a drug-induced lupus-like syndrome. Methysergide therapy also has been implicated as a cause of constrictive pericarditis.

Diagnosis			
History	General		• Constrictive pericarditis presents with a myriad of symptoms, making a diagnosis based solely on clinical history unlikely.
	Dyspnea		• Dyspnea tends to be the most common presenting symptom and occurs in virtually all patients.
	Fatigue		• Fatigue and orthopnea are commonly seen.
	Edema		• Lower-extremity edema and abdominal swelling and discomfort are other common symptoms.
	Ascites		• The initial history may be more suggestive of liver disease (cryptogenic cirrhosis) than pericardial constriction because of the predominance of findings related to the venous system (i.e. ascites, peripheral edema etc
Physical examination	General		• Constriction should be considered in the presence of otherwise unexplained jugular venous distention, pleural effusion, hepatomegaly, or ascites.
	Increased jugular venous pressure		• Elevated jugular venous pressures almost are always present. • The apical impulse often is not palpable, and the patient may have distant or muffled heart sounds.
	Pericardial knock		• A pericardial knock, which corresponds with the sudden cessation of ventricular filling early in diastole, occurs in approximately half the cases and may be mistaken for an S_3 gallop. • A knock is of higher frequency than an S_3 gallop and occurs slightly earlier in diastole.
	Pulsus paradoxus		• Pulsus paradoxus is a variable finding and, if present, rarely exceeds 10 mm Hg unless a concomitant pericardial effusion exists with an abnormally elevated pressure .
	Kussmaul sign	•	The Kussmaul sign (i.e., elevation of systemic venous pressures with inspiration) is a common nonspecific finding, but this sign also is observed in patients with right ventricular failure, restrictive cardiomyopathy, right ventricular infarction, and tricuspid stenosis.
	Hepatomegaly		• Hepatomegaly with prominent hepatic pulsations can be detected in as many as 70% of patients.

Diagnostic Tests	
Laboratory testing	• Serum BNP levels are nearly normal or mildly elevated in patients with constrictive physiology of heart failure and grossly elevated in patients with restrictive physiology, despite nearly identical clinical and hemodynamic presentation. • Elevations in both conjugated and unconjugated bilirubin levels, and elevated levels of hepatocellular function tests related to hepatic congestion.
Chest radiography	• May show pericardial calcification which is found in 20% to 30% of patients; however, it is not specific and does not prove pericardial constriction • Pleural effusions are common.
Echocardiography	• Two-dimensional echocardiography may show evidence of right-sided pressure overload, such as atrial septal shifting to the left with inspiration, or dilated inferior and superior vena cavae and hepatic veins. • Pericardial imaging by echocardiography is not sensitive and is not considered a reliable technique to visualize the pericardium. • Respiratory variations of diastolic (transmitral) blood flow help to differentiate between constrictive pericarditis and restrictive cardiomyopathy (RCM). A pattern of respiratory variation, with a diminished peak transmitral diastolic flow during inspiration, is characteristic of pericardial constriction but not of RCM. • Since myocardial relaxation itself is preserved in pure constrictive pericarditis, the early relaxation myocardial velocity on tissue Doppler imaging (E_a, also known as E_m) is normal, whereas it is abnormal with restriction (when intrinsic myocardial disease is present).
High resolution computed tomography (CT)	• The parietal pericardium can be visualized well using high-resolution CT. • Pericardial thickening of more than 4 mm assists in differentiating constrictive disease from restrictive cardiomyopathy, and a thickening of more than 6 mm adds even more specificity for constriction.
Magnetic resonance (MR) imaging	• As can be done with CT scanning, an MRI can be used to measure the pericardium for thickness, calcification, and distribution of abnormalities.

Cardiac catheterization	• Elevated left and right ventricular diastolic pressures equalized within 5 mm Hg. • Right ventricular systolic pressure < 55 mm Hg • Mean right arterial pressure > 15 mm Hg • Right ventricular end-diastolic pressure greater than one third of the right ventricular systolic pressure (narrow pulse pressure)

Treatment

General information		• Medical management is generally ineffective.
Pharmaco-therapy	Diuretics	• Diuretics are commonly used to relieve congestion if ventricular filling pressures are clinically elevated. However, this may decrease cardiac output and requires careful monitoring.
	No β-Blockers or calcium channel blockers	• In general, β-Blockers and calcium channel blockers should be avoided because the sinus tachycardia that commonly occurs in constrictive pericarditis is compensatory in nature (maintaining cardiac output in a setting of fixed stroke volume).
	Anticoagulation	• Patients with a history of embolization or atrial fibrillation should be anticoagulated
	Cardiac transplantation	• Can be considered in highly selected patients with refractory symptoms in idiopathic or familial RCM and amyloidosis
Invasive therapy	Complete pericardectomy	• Is the definitive therapy and is potentially curative

3.8.5   Takotsubo Cardiomyopathy (TCM)

Epidemiology

- *Takotsubo* cardiomyopathy (also called stress induced cardiomyopathy, apical ballooning, or broken heart syndrome) is characterized by acute, reversible left ventricular dysfunction in a characteristic distribution, which does not correlate with epicardial coronary artery blood supply.
- The characteristic appearances seen initially on contrast angiography are a ballooned apical segment and a hypercontractile basal portion of the left ventricle.
- The Japanese word *takotsubo* means "octopus pot," which resembles the shape of the left ventricle during systole on imaging studies with this condition.
- This condition is responsible for 1% to 2% of admissions for acute coronary syndrome in industrialized countries.
- *Takotsubo* cardiomyopathy mainly affects postmenopausal women and is unusual in men.
- Symptoms seem to be triggered by psychological or physical stress (such as death of a family member, alcohol or drug withdrawal, acute somatic disorder, or major surgery).
- An increased incidence has been reported after natural disasters such as earthquakes.

Pathophysiology

- The pathophysiology of *takotsubo* cardiomyopathy includes endocrine, hormonal, neuropsychological, and microvascular factors.
- The most commonly accepted mechanism for *takotsubo* cardiomyopathy (TCM) is stress-induced catecholamine release, with toxicity to and subsequent stunning of the myocardium.
- The apical portions of the left ventricle have the highest concentration of sympathetic innervation found in the heart and may explain why excess catecholamines may selectively affect its function.

Causes

- Idiopathic
- Emotional or physical stressor
- Stressors include learning of a death in the family, natural disasters, motor vehicle collisions, exacerbation of a chronic medical illness, newly diagnosed significant medical condition, surgery, intensive care unit stay, and use of or withdrawal from illicit drugs
- TCM has been reported after near drowning episodes.

Diagnosis		
History	Dyspnea Chest pain	• The most common presenting symptoms are chest pain and dyspnea. • Palpitations, syncope, and rarely, cardiogenic shock have been reported • History of a preceding emotionally or physically stressful trigger event
Physical examination	General	• **Patients may have the clinical appearance of having acute coronary syndrome or acute congestive heart failure.**
	Arrythmias	• Both tachy- and bradyarrhythmias may be seen
	Lung rales	• May be present in the setting of acute pulmonary edema
	Low blood pressure and signs of hypoperfusion	• Suggestive of cardiogenic shock
	Signs of thromboembolism	• May be evident

Diagnostic Tests	
Laboratory testing	• Cardiac markers, specifically troponin I and T, are elevated in 90% of patients with *takotsubo* cardiomyopathy • Brain natriuretic peptide (BNP) level is frequently elevated, especially in patients with overt heart failure.
Chestradiography	• May show pulmonary edema
ECG	• May show ST-segment elevation (67% to 75%) and T-wave inversion (61%)
Echocardiography	• Two-dimensional echocardiography shows hypokinesis or akinesis of the mid and apical segments of the left ventricle. • Regional wall motion abnormalities extend beyond the distribution of any single coronary artery.
Magnetic resonance (MR) imaging	• Can differentiate *takotsubo* cardiomyopathy, characterized by the absence of delayed gadolinium hyperenhancement, from myocardial infarction and myocarditis in which there is presence of delayed hyperenhancement
Cardiac catheterization	• Normal or nonobstructive coronary artery disease
Left ventriculography	• Perhaps the best imaging modality to demonstrate the pathognomonic wall motion and to evaluate ejection fraction

Treatment		
General information		• Because *takotsubo* cardiomyopathy (TCM) mimics acute coronary syndrome (ACS) and no initial ECG finding reliably differentiates *takotsubo* cardiomyopathy from an ST-segment elevation myocardial infarction (STEMI), clinicians should follow established protocols for managing patients with ACS. • The left ventricular abnormality usually reverses spontaneously in days or weeks.
Pharmaco-therapy	Diuretics	• Patients in acute heart failure may require diuresis.
	ACE inhibitors and β- Blockers	• Standard therapy for left ventricular dysfunction should be initiated, including use of angiotensin-converting enzyme inhibitors and β-Blockers.
	Anticoagulation	• Anticoagulants may be used to treat or prevent left ventricular apical thrombus.
	Caution with inotropes	• Hyperkinetic basal segment may cause outflow obstruction, and inotropes may exacerbate the problem and should be used with caution.
Invasive therapy	Intraaortic balloon pump	• Insertion of an intra-aortic balloon pump is recommended in those with cardiogenic shock.

3.9 Arrhythmias

3.9.1 Atrial Flutter/Fibrillation

Epidemiology

- Atrial fibrillation (AF) is the most common tachyarrhythmia.
- Atrial flutter (AFL) is the second most common tachyarrhythmia, after atrial fibrillation.
- Atrial flutter is characterized by a macro re-entrant arrhythmia with atrial rates between 240-300 beats per minute.
- Atrial flutter affects approximately 88 out of 100 000 new patients each year.
- Atrial fibrillation affects more than 2.2 million Americans and almost 5% of the population older than 69 years.

Pathophysiology

- Atrial flutter is caused by a re-entrant circuit that is confined to the right atrium (RA).
- The impulses travel through the atrial septum, then across the right atrium, then inferiorly through the right atrium free wall, and then back across through an isthmus bounded by the coronary sinus os and the tricuspid valve annulus.
- This isthmus also is called the atrial flutter isthmus and is the target for radiofrequency catheter ablation of atrial flutter.
- The multiple wavelet hypothesis for atrial fibrillation proposes that fractionation of wavefronts propagating through the atria results in self-perpetuating "daughter" wavelets and multiple reentry circuits
- Atrial fibrillation appears to require both an initiating event and a permissive atrial substrate.

Causes

- Hypertension
- Valvular heart disease
- Left ventricular hypertrophy
- Coronary artery disease with or without depressed left ventricular function
- Pericarditis
- Pulmonary embolism
- Hyperthyroidism
- Diabetes mellitus
- Post-cardiac surgery
- Acute coronary syndrome
- Drug use: stimulants, alcohol, and cocaine can trigger atrial flutter or fibrillation
- Cerebrovascular events such as subarachnoid hemorrhage or stroke

Diagnosis		
History		• Palpitations (most common symptom) • Fatigue • Dyspnea on exertion • Less common symptoms include angina, profound dyspnea, or syncope. • Thromboembolic events, i.e. stroke, TIA
Physical examination	Heart rate changes	• Tachycardia: heart rate in atrial flutter is often approximately 150 beats per minute because of a 2:1 AV block • Irregularly irregular heart rate is seen in atrial fibrillation
	Lung rales	• In patients with heart failure

Diagnostic Tests		
Laboratory testing		• TSH • Serum electrolytes • Digitalis levels
ECG	Atrial flutter	• The ECG usually demonstrates a regular rhythm, with P waves that can appear sawtoothed, also called flutter waves. • Since the atrioventricular (AV) node cannot conduct at the same rate as the atrial activity, one commonly sees some form of conduction block, typically 2:1 or 4:1. • This block also may be variable and cause atrial flutter to appear as an irregular rhythm. • Atrial flutter can conduct to the ventricle in a 1:1 fashion, producing a ventricular rate of 300 beats per minute in patients with the pre-excitation syndrome.
	Atrial fibrillation	• Absence of sinus P waves • Rapid oscillations or F waves that vary in amplitude, frequency, and shape • An irregular ventricular response
Echocardiography		• Assists in diagnosing valvular heart disease, left ventricular hypertrophy (LVH), and pericardial disease
Holter monitor		• Can be used to help identify arrhythmias in patients with non-specific symptoms, identify triggers, and detect associated atrial arrhythmias

Treatment

General goals of treatment for both atrial flutter and fibrillation are	• Control of the ventricular rate (see Rate control) • Restoration of sinus rhythm (see Rhythm control) • Prevention and decreased frequency or duration of recurrent episodes • Prevention of thromboembolic complications

If Patient is Hemodynamically Unstable:

Emergency cardioversion	• If the patient is unstable (eg., hypotension, heart failure, angina), synchronous direct-current (DC) cardioversion is the initial treatment of choice. • Cardioversion for flutter may be successful with energies as low as 25 Joules, but since 100 Joules is virtually always successful, this may be a reasonable initial shock strength. • If the electrical shock results in atrial fibrillation (AF), a second shock at a higher energy level is used to restore normal sinus rhythm (NSR).

If Patient is Hemodynamically Stable:

Rate control	Adenosine	Produces transient AV block and can be used to reveal flutter waves
	β-Blockers	Should be considered first line agents for rate control
	Cacium channel blockers	i.e. verapamil or diltiazem also may be appropriate initial treatment
	Digoxin	Digoxin may be used as adjunctive therapy for rate control, although less effective than β-Blockers or calcium channel blockers
	Caution with certain conditions	A history of **Wolff-Parkinson-White (WPW) syndrome** or evidence of **ventricular preexcitation should be determined** because agents that act exclusively at the level of the AV node may enhance accessory pathway conduction. Procainamide is the initial drug of choice for atrial flutter or fibrillation in patients with WPW syndrome.
Rhythm control (drugs)	Dofetilide	Effective in 70% to 80% of patients
	Ibutilide	Is effective, **converting recent-onset atrial flutter** to sinus rhythm in approximately 60% of patients with a single infusion.
	Type IC anti-arrhythmic agents	Ppropafenone (450-600 mg) or flecainide (200-300 mg) have also been shown to be effective in **converting recent-onset atrial fibrillation** to sinus rhythm.
	Amio-, drone-darone, sotalol	Can be used for patients with ischemic or structural heart disease

| Rhythm control (invasive therapies) | Radiofrequency catheter ablation | Is now the **long-term treatment of choice** in patients with **symptomatic atrial flutter**. |
| | Surgical MAZE procedure or catheter-based pulmonary vein ablation | Options for patients with atrial fibrillation who have failed medical therapy or are not considered candidates for such therapy |

Thromboembolic Prophylaxis

Indicated in all patients with atrial flutter and fibrillation based on the CHADS$_2$ score

CHADS$_2$-Score

- The CHADS$_2$ stroke risk stratification scheme should be used as an initial, rapid, and easy-to-remember means of assessing stroke risk.
- The CHADS$_2$ index uses a point system to determine yearly thromboembolic risk.
- **Two points** are assigned for a **history of stroke or TIA**, and **one point** is given **for age over 75 or a history of hypertension, diabetes, or heart failure.**

| CHADS$_2$ | ≤ 1 | Use aspirin 81-325 mg daily |
| CHADS$_2$ | > 1 | Use warfarin ,with target INR 2.0 - 3.0 |

CHA$_2$DS$_2$-VASc-Score

- The risk factor-based approach for patients with non-valvular AF can also be expressed as an acronym, CHA2DS2-VASc [congestive heart failure, hypertension, age ≥ 75 y (doubled), diabetes, stroke (doubled), vascular disease, age 65-74 y, and sex category (female)]
- This scheme is based on a point system in which 2 points are assigned for a history of stroke or TIA, or age ≥ 75 y; and 1 point each is assigned for age 65-74 years, a history of hypertension, diabetes, recent cardiac failure, vascular disease (myocardial infarction, complex aortic plaque, and PAD, including prior revascularization, amputation due to PAD, or angiographic evidence of PAD, etc.), and female sex.
- This system extends the CHADS$_2$ scheme by considering additional stroke risk factors that may influence a decision whether or not to anticoagulate.

ECG-Example: Atrial Fibrillation

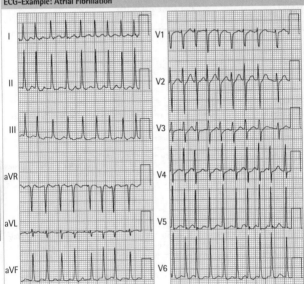

3.9.2 Ventricular Tachycardia

Epidemiology

- Ventricular tachycardia (VT) is defined as three or more beats of ventricular origin in succession at a rate greater than 100 beats per minute.
- The hemodynamic consequences of VT depend largely on the presence or absence or myocardial dysfunction (such as might result from ischemia or infarction) and on the rate of VT.
- Ventricular tachycardia can be referred to as sustained or nonsustained.
  - Sustained VT refers to an episode that lasts at least 30 seconds and generally requires termination by antiarrhythmia drugs, antitachycardia pacing techniques or electrical cardioversion.
  - Nonsustained VT suggests that the episodes are short (three beats or longer) and terminate spontaneously.

Pathophysiology

- The most common setting for VT is ischemic heart disease, in which myocardial scar is the substrate for electrical reentry.
- It can also be seen in nonischemic cardiomyopathies, ion channel abnormalities, and other conditions in which cardiac function and structure are normal.
- Hemodynamic collapse is more likely when underlying left ventricular dysfunction is present or with very rapid rates.
- When the ventricular activation sequence is constant, the electrocardiographic pattern remains the same, and the rhythm is called monomorphic VT.
- Monomorphic VT is most commonly seen in patients with underlying structural heart disease.
- Polymorphic VT occurs when the ventricular activation sequence varies.

Causes

- Myocardial infarction	- Congenital or acquired long QT syndrome
- Myocardial scar	- Arrhythmogenic right ventricular dysplasia
- Coronary artery disease	- Congenital heart diseases
- Cardiomyopathies	

Diagnosis

History	Palpitations	• The main symptoms of VT are palpitation, lightheadedness, and syncope from diminished cerebral perfusion
	Lightheadedness	• Syncope is more common in the setting of structural heart disease.
	Syncope	
	Chest pain	Chest pain may be due to ischemia or the rhythm.

Physical examination	Tachycardia	
	Signs of ↓ perfusion	May be present, including diminished level of consciousness, pallor, and diaphoresis
	Cannon a waves	May be observed in jugular venous pulse if the atria are in sinus rhythm
	S_1 variation	May vary in intensity due to AV dissociation

Diagnostic Tests	
Laboratory testing	• Include electrolyte levels in an acute evaluation. Hypokalemia is a common VT trigger and is commonly seen in patients taking diuretics. • Check cardiac enzyme levels if clinical symptoms or signs of ischemia are present
ECG	• Rate > 100 beats per minute and usually not faster than 200 beats per minute. • Rhythm is usually regular but may be irregular. • Atrioventricular dissociation • QRS axis between -90° and +180° or - 180° • The width of the QRS is 0.12 s or greater. • The QRS morphology is often bizarre, with notching. • The ST segment and T wave are usually opposite in polarity to the QRS (discordance).
Echocardiography	Assists in diagnosing LV function and other structural heart disease
Coronary angiography	May be indicated to assess for coronary obstruction

Treatment	

If Patient is Hemodynamically Unstable

Emergency cardioversion	• Ventricular tachycardia (VT) associated with loss of consciousness or hypotension is a medical emergency requiring immediate cardioversion • 100-to 200J biphasic cardioversion

If Patient is Hemodynamically Stable

If no evidence for coronary ischemia or infarction is present, then rhythm conversion may be attempted with intravenous medication.

Rhythm conversion (with intravenous medication)	Amiodarone	150 mg IV infused over 10 min, followed by 1 mg/min constant infusion for 6 h, then maintenance infusion at 0.5 mg/min; oral dosing generally 400 mg/d following load
	Lidocaine	1-1.5 mg/kg IV push, followed by 0.5-0.75 mg/kg IV push to a maximum of 3 mg/kg; Continuous 1-4 mg/min infusion should be started after arrhythmia is suppressed

If Medical Therapy is Unsuccessful	
Synchronized cardioversion	50-200 J (monophasic) following sedation is appropriate
Endocardial catheter ablation	May be used in idiopathic monomorphic VT
Implantable cardioverter-defibrillator (ICD)	Evaluation for ICD-implantation is indicated after resuscitation, and cardiac electrophysiology should be consulted

ECG-Example: Ventricular Tachycardia

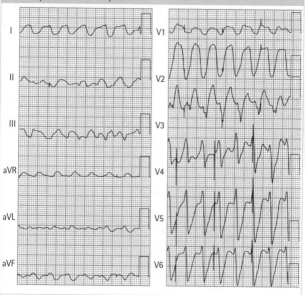

3.9.3   Ventricular Fibrillation

Epidemiology

- Ventricular fibrillation (VF) is a potentially fatal, uncoordinated series of very rapid, ineffective contractions of the ventricles caused by many chaotic electrical impulses.
- VF causes loss of consciousness in seconds, and if the disorder is not immediately treated, is fatal.
- VF is the most commonly identified arrhythmia in cardiac arrest patients.
- Cardiopulmonary resuscitation (CPR) must be started within a few minutes, and it must be followed by defibrillation (an electrical shock delivered to the chest) to restore normal heart rhythm.
- Sudden cardiac death accounts for approximately 300 000 deaths per year in the United States, of which 75% to 80% are due to VF.

Pathophysiology

- VF occurs in a variety of clinical situations but is most often associated with coronary artery disease (CAD).
- VF may be due to acute myocardial infarction or ischemia, or it may occur in the setting of chronic infarct scar.

Causes

• Myocardial infarction	• Myocarditis
• Electrical shock	• WPW with atrial fibrillation
• Drowning	• Brugada syndrome
• Drugs	• Arrhythmogenic RV cardiomyopathy/ dysplasia
• Severe hypokalemia	• Long QT syndrome
• Hypoxia	
• Cardiomyopathy	

Diagnosis

History	Chest pain	• Obtaining a thorough history from the patient, family members, or other witnesses is necessary to obtain insight into the events surrounding the episode of VF.
		• A history of LV impairment (LV ejection fraction [LVEF] < 30% to 35%) is the single greatest risk factor for sudden death from VF.

Physical exami-nation	Assess cardiac arrest score	ED SBP greater than 90 mm Hg	1 point
		ED SBP less than 90 mm Hg	0 points
		Time to ROSC less than 25 minutes	1 point
		Time to ROSC more than 25 minutes	0 points
		Neurologically responsive	1 point
		Comatose	0 points
		Maximum score = 3 points	
		Patients with a score of 3 points can be expected to have approximately 90% chance of neurologic recovery and an 82% chance of survival to discharge. Severe anoxic encephalopathy in patients with scores of 0, 1, or 2 suggests the use of conservative management with empiric supportive and medical therapy. ED = end-diastolic; ROSC = return of spontaneous circulation; SBP = systolic blood pressure	

Diagnostic Tests	
Laboratory testing	• Include electrolyte levels in an acute evaluation. Severe metabolic acidosis, hypokalemia, hyperkalemia, hypocalcemia, and hypomagnesemia are some of the conditions that can increase the risk for arrhythmia and sudden death. • Check cardiac enzyme levels if clinical symptoms or signs of ischemia are present.
ECG	• There are no normal-looking QRS complexes. • Bizarre, irregular, random waveform • No clearly identifiable QRS complexes or P waves • Wandering baseline
Echocardiography	Assists in assessing LV function and other structrural heart disease
Coronary angiography	May be indicated to assess for acute coronary occlusion

Treatment

In the event of cardiac arrest		• Immediate implementation of ACLS guidelines is indicated
External electrical defibrillation (remains the most successful treatment of VF)	Deliver 1 defibrillation shock to the patient	• Automated External Defibrillator (AED), by specific; monophasic adult, 200 J; child, 2 J/kg (or equivalent biphasic energy) • Biphasic defibrillation has a number of advantages over monophasic defibrillation including increased likelihood of defibrillation success for a given shocking energy
	Before any defibrillation	• Remove all patches and ointments from the chest wall because they create a risk of fire or explosion.
	Treat underlying provocative abnormalities	• MI, hypovolemia, hemorrhagic shock, anoxia/hypoxia, pneumothorax/hemothorax, hypercalcemia, drug overdose (narcotic, tricyclic antidepressant, cocaine, barbiturate), carbon monoxide poisoning, hyperkalemia, etc
Consider antiarrhythmic agents (to give during CPR, before or after the shock)	Amiodarone	• 300 mg IV/IO once, then consider additional 150 mg IV/IO once
	or Lidocaine	• 1-1.5 mg/kg IV/IO first dose, then 0.5-0.75 mg/kg IV/IO, maximum 3 doses or 3 mg/kg
	Consider magnesium sulfate	• Loading dose 1-2 g IV/IO for *torsades de pointes*
Implantable cardioverter-defibrillator (ICD)		• Evaluation for Implantable cardioverter-defibrillator (ICD) implantation is indicated • Most survivors of VF should receive ICD.

3.9.4 High-grade and Complete AV Block

Epidemiology

- Atrioventricular (AV) block occurs when the atrial depolarization fails to reach the ventricles
- High-grade AV Block
  - High-grade AV block consists of multiple P waves in a row that are not conducted
  - The conduction ratio can be 3:1 or more and the PR interval of conducted beats is constant
  - It is different from complete AV block in that the P waves that conduct to the QRS complexes occur at fixed intervals
- For complete AV block, no relationship exists between the P waves and QRS complexes
  - Complete heart block (CHB) is diagnosed when no supraventricular impulses are conducted to the ventricles
  - P waves on the ECG reflect a sinus node rhythm independent from QRS complexes
- AV blocks occur more frequently in people older than 70 years, especially in those who have structural heart disease.

Pathophysiology

- High-grade AV block is caused by conduction disturbances in the AV node or the His-Purkinje system.
- In most cases of complete AV block, an escape rhythm originates from the ventricles, with wide QRS complexes at a low regular rate of 30-40 beats per minute.

Causes

- Myocardial ischemia/ infarction
- Degenerative changes in the AV node or bundle branches
- Drugs (digitalis glycosides, b-Blockers, calcium channel blockers, other antiarrhythmic agents)
- Infiltrative myocardial diseases (sarcoidosis, myxedema, hemochromatosis)
- Endocarditis and other infections such as Lyme disease
- Surgical (e.g. aortic valve replacement, congenital defect repair)

Diagnosis

History	General	• May occasionally be asymptomatic
	Lightheadedness, syncope	• Fatigue, dizziness, lightheadedness, presyncope, and syncope are reported most commonly. • Chest pain, dyspnea, confusion, pulmonary edema may be seen.
Physical examination	Bradycardia	
	Cannon a waves	• May be observed in the jugular venous pulse
	S_1 intensity	• A variable intensity S_1 may be heard.
	Signs of systemic hypoperfusion	• Assess signs of systemic hypoperfusion, i.e. altered mental status, hypotension

Diagnostic Tests	
Laboratory testing	• Levels of electrolytes and drugs (e.g. digitalis) should be checked in the case of second-degree or third-degree AV block when suspicion of increased potassium level or drug toxicity exists. • Check cardiac enzyme levels if clinical symptoms or signs of ischemia are present.
ECG	• Complete lack of conduction (no P waves cause a QRS complex) characterizes third-degree heart block. • If complete AV block exists, then the R-R interval is very regular; therefore, before diagnosing third-degree AV block, the R-R interval should be either marched out or measured. • If high-grade AV block exists without complete heart block, then some irregularity may occur during intervals following conducted P waves.
Echocardiography	• Assists in assessing LV function and other structrural heart disease
Coronary angiography	• May be indicated to assess for acute coronary occlusion

Treatment	
General information	• The first medical treatment for heart block is the withdrawal of any potentially aggravating or causative medications. • Initial efforts should focus on assessing the need for temporary pacing and initiating the pacing.
Consider pacemaker in patients with	• Symptomatic bradycardia • Documented periods of asystole greater than or equal to 3.0 seconds or any escape rate less than 40 bpm in awake, symptom-free patients • Neuromuscular diseases with AV block, such as myotonic muscular dystrophy, Kearns-Sayre syndrome, Erb dystrophy (limb-girdle), and peroneal muscular atrophy, with or without symptoms, because unpredictable progression of AV conduction disease may occur • Postoperative AV block that is not expected to resolve after cardiac surgery

ECG-Example: AV-Block, Second Degree

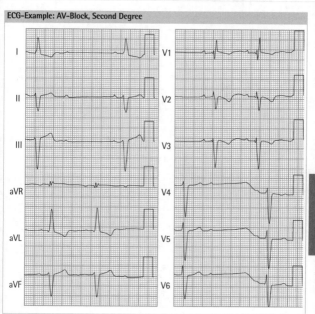

ECG-Example: AV-Block, Third Degree

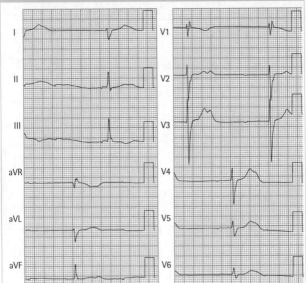

3.10 Heart Failure

3.10.1 Generall Information

Definition	The inability of the heart to fill with or eject blood sufficient to meet metabolic demands as a result of either a structural or functional disorder of the myocardium, endocardium, or pericardium.
Pathophysiology	The majority of patients with heart failure have dysfunction of the left ventricular myocardium, leading to a change in geometry (dilatation) and sometimes structure (hypertrophy), a process known as remodeling.
Clinical manifestations	Dyspnea, fatigue, impaired functional capacity, and fluid retention leading to peripheral and/or pulmonary edema.
Epidemiology	• According to the AHA, there are 5 million people in the US who have heart failure (HF) and 550 000 new diagnoses of HF made annually. • Heart failure accounts for over 1 million hospitalizations each year and is the leading cause of hospitalization among Medicare recipients.
Risk factors	• Advancing age • Coronary artery disease • Hypertension • Myocardial infarction • Diabetes mellitus • Valvular disease	• Obesity • Excessive alcohol intake • Smoking • Dyslipidemia • Sleep-disordered breathing • Chronic kidney disease

3.10.2 Neurohormonal Mechanisms of Heart Failure

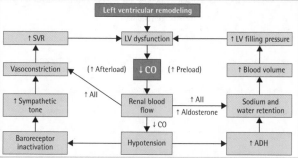

All = angiotensin II; ADH = antidiuretic hormone; CO = cardiac output; LV = left ventricle; SVR = systemic vascular resistance; RAAS = renin-angiotensin-aldosterone system.

Angiotensin II Effects	Aldosterone Effects
• ↑ Water and sodium reabsorption, ↑ADH release, ↑Release of aldosterone from adrenal cortex • Myocyte necrosis, fibroblast proliferation, and myocardial fibrosis ⇒ cardiac remodeling	• ↑ Water and sodium reabsorption • Myocyte necrosis, fibroblast proliferation, and myocardial fibrosis ⇒ cardiac remodeling with possible dilatation

- Falling cardiac output leads to decreased renal blood flow and activation of the RAAS.
- The compensatory mechanisms triggered by renin, aldosterone, and angiotensin II are designed to combat the effects of decreased arterial filling pressure; all cause water reabsorption out of proportion to sodium reabsorption, leading to hyponatremia.
- Hypotension resulting from a further fall in cardiac output activates the CNS release of ADH.
- Inactivation of baroreceptors enhances sympathetic tone and vasoconstriction.
- As cardiac output, renal blood flow, and systemic blood pressure remain reduced, these mechanisms continue to increase preload and afterload, leading to further reduction in cardiac output and left ventricular dysfunction.

3.10.3   Causes of Nonischemic Cardiomyopathy

Infiltrative diseases	• Amyloidosis	
Intracellular storage diseases	• Hemochromatosis • Glycogen storage diseases	• Fabry disease • Niemann–Pick disease
Endomyocardial diseases	• Endomyocardial fibrosis	• Loeffler endocarditis
Granulomatous diseases	• Sarcoidosis	
Endocrine disorders	• Diabetes mellitus • Hyper- or hypothyroidism • Hyperparathyroidism	• Pheochromocytoma • Acromegaly
Nutritional deficiencies	• Beriberi • Scurvy • Pellagra	• Carnitine deficiency • Selenium deficiency
Collagen Vascular diseases	• Rheumatoid arthritis • Systemic lupus erythematosus	• Dermatomyositis • Scleroderma • Polyarteritis nodosa
Chemotherapeutic agents	• Anthracyclines (doxorubicin, daunorubicin)	• Cyclophosphamide • Radiation
Infections	• HIV • Chagas disease (T. cruzi)	• Lyme disease
Toxins	• Alcohol abuse	

3.10.4 Progression of Heart Failure

STAGE A	STAGE B	STAGE C	STAGE D
At high risk for HF but without structural heart disease or symptoms of HF	Structural heart disease but without signs or symptoms of HF	Structural heart disease with prior or current symptoms of HF	Refractory HF requiring specialized interventions

e.g. Patients with:	e.g. Patients with:	e.g. Patients with:	e.g. Patients:
• hypertension • atherosclerotic disease • diabetes • obesity • metabolic syndrome or Patients: • using cardiotoxins • with FHx CM	• previous MI • LV remodeling including LVH and low EF • asymptomatic valvular disease	• known structural heart disease and • shortness of breath and fatigue, reduced exercise tolerance	• who have marked symptoms at rest despite max. medical Tx (e.g. those who are recurrently hospitalized or cannot be safely discharged from the hospital without specialized interventions

Structural heart disease → Development of symptoms of HF → Refractory symptoms of HF at rest →

THERAPY	THERAPY	THERAPY	THERAPY
Goals: • Treat hypertension • Encourage smoking cessation • Treat lipid disorders • Encourage regular exercise • Discourage alcohol intake, illicit drug use • Control metabolic syndrome **Drugs:** ACEI or ARB in appropriate patients for vascular disease or diabetes	**Goals:** • All measures under Stage A **Drugs:** • ACEI or ARB in appropriate patients, BB in appropriate patients **Devices in selected patients:** • Implantable defibrillators	**Goals:** • All measures under Stages A and B • Dietary salt restriction **Drugs for routine use:** • Diuretics for fluid retention, ACEI, BB **Drugs in selected patients:** • Aldosterone antagonist, ARBs, Digitalis, hydralazine, nitrates **Devices in selected patients:** • Biventricular pacing • Implantable Defibrillators	**Goals:** • Appropriate measures under Stages A, B, C • Decision re: appropriate level of care **Options:** • Compassionate end of life care/hospice • Extraordinary measures • Heart transplant • Chronic inotropes • Permanent mechanical support • Experimental surgery or drugs

BB = Betablocker, FHx CM = family history of cardiomyopathy; reprinted from the Journal of the American College of Cardiology, 53 (15), 2009 Focused Update Incorporated Into the ACC/AHA 2005 Guidelines for the Diagnosis and Management of Heart Failure in Adults, Hunt SA, et al. , e1-e90. Copyright 2009, with permission from the American College of Cardiology Foundation and the American Heart Association, Inc. Published by Elsevier Inc.

3.10.5 New York Heart Association Classification of Heart Failure

NYHA Class	Symptoms
Class 1	Patient is asymptomatic
Class 2	Patient is symptomatic with ordinary level of exertion
Class 3	Patient is symptomatic with less than ordinary level of exertion
Class 4	Patient is symptomatic at rest

3.10.6 Assessment/Treatment of Acute Decompensated Heart Failure

	Congestion at Rest	
	No	Yes
No	**Warm and dry:** – Compensated patient	**Warm and wet:** – Diuretics – Ultrafiltration
Yes	**Cold and dry:** – Fluids – Inotropes	**Cold and wet:** – Inotropes – Vasodilators

(Low Perfusion at Rest)

PCWP − 18 + PCWP

Signs and symptoms of congestion:
- Orthopnea/PND
- Jugular venous distension
- Hepatomegaly
- Edema
- Rales
- Elevated estimated pulmonary artery pressure (loud P_2 and RV lift)
- Hepatojugular reflux
- S_3 heart sound

Possible evidence of low perfusion:
- Narrow pulse pressure
- Sleepy/obtunded
- Low serum sodium
- Elevated liver function tests
- Cool extremities
- Hypotension with use of ACEIs
- Renal dysfunction

PCWP = pulmonary capillary wedge pressure; PND= paroxysmal nocturnal dyspnea

3.10.7 PRIDE Acute Congestive Heart Failure (CHF) Score

Predictor	Points	Predictor	Points
Elevated NT-proBNP	4	Current loop diuretic use	1
Interstitial edema on CXR	2	Age > 75 years	1
Orthopnea	2	Rales on lung examination	1
Absence of fever	2	Absence of cough	1

CXR = chest radiography; BNP = brain natriuretic peptide; **Scoring: Add relevant points to arrive at a total score; a total score of 7 has a high predictive accuracy for the diagnosis of acute CHF.** Reprinted with permission from Baggish AL, et al., A Clinical and Biochemical Critical Pathway for the Evaluation of Patients With Suspected Acute Congestive Heart Failure. The ProBNP Investigation of Dyspnea in the Emergency Department (PRIDE) AlgorithmCrit Pathw Cardiol. 2004; 3(4):171–6. Copyright 2004 by Lippincott Williams & Wilkins. Published by Wolters Kluwer Health.

3.10.8 Clinical Evaluation/Triage for Patients with Suspected Acute CHF

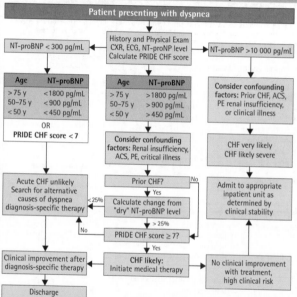

CHF = congestive heart failure; ACS = acute coronary syndrome; PE = pulmonary embolus
Reprinted with permission from Baggish AL, et al., A Clinical and Biochemical Critical Pathway for the Evaluation of Patients With Suspected Acute Congestive Heart Failure. The ProBNP Investigation of Dyspnea in the Emergency Department (PRIDE) Algorithm *Crit Pathw Cardiol.* 2004; 3(4):171-6. Copyright 2004 by Lippincott Williams & Wilkins. Published by Wolters Kluwer Health.

3.10.9 Initial Evaluation of Patients with Heart Failure

Patient History	Laboratory Data
Perform careful assessment of the patient's history with an emphasis on heart failure risk factors (see risk factors section). Questions you should ask: • Can you carry out daily activities without difficulty? • How far can you walk before having to stop because you are short of breath? • How far could you walk 6 months ago? • Do you ever wake up in the middle of the night feeling as if you are smothering and cannot breathe?	• Complete blood count • Complete metabolic panel • Liver function tests • Urinalysis • Lipid panel • Fasting plasma glucose • Hemoglobin A1C • Thyroid function tests • BNP or NT-proBNP

Physical	Other Studies
• Functional status • Orthostatic changes • Volume status • Body-mass index • Blood pressure • Weight and height	• 12-lead ECG • Chest radiography • Transthoracic echocardiogram to evaluate ejection fraction, left ventricular size, and wall thickness • Coronary angiography should be performed on patients with newly diagnosed heart failure to evaluate for ischemic etiology

Family History	
• Premature coronary disease • Sudden cardiac death • Myopathy	• Conduction disturbances • Tachyarrhythmias

3.10.10 Indications for Implantable Cardiac Defibrillator for Primary Prevention

NYHA Class	Cardiomyopathy Type	Ejection Fraction
1	Ischemic, at least 40 days post-MI	< 30%
2	Ischemic, at least 40 days post-MI	≤ 35%
	Nonischemic	≤ 35%
3	Ischemic, at least 40 days post-MI	≤ 35%
	Nonischemic	≤ 35%

3.10.11 Indications for Cardiac Resynchronization Therapy (CRT)*

NYHA Class	Ejection Fraction	QRS Length	Other Required Criteria
3 or 4 (ambulating)	≤ 35%	> 120 ms	Normal sinus rhythm and currently on maximal medical therapy

Table 3.10.10 and 3.10.11 reprinted from the Journal of the American College of Cardiology, 51 (21), Epstein AE, et al. , ACC/AHA/HRS 2008 Guidelines for Device-Based Therapy of Cardiac Rhythm Abnormalities, e1-e62, Copyright 2008, with permission from the American College of Cardiology Foundation, the American Heart Association, Inc., and the Heart Rhythm Society. Published by Elsevier Inc.

3.10.12 Heart Failure with Preserved Left Ventricular Function

Symptoms	Patient Profile	Common Etiology
Similar to patients with ↓ LV ejection fraction: • Dyspnea • Pulmonary edema • Fatigue • ↓ exercise tolerance	• Older patients • Females • Non-African American • History of hypertension • History of diabetes mellitus	• Restrictive cardiomyopathy • Obstructive and non-obstructive hypertrophic cardiomyopathy • Infiltrative cardiomyopathy • Often, no identifiable etiology

Diagnostic Features

- Increased LV end-diastolic pressure in patients with heart failure symptoms
- Preserved left ventricular function
- No valvular abnormalities

Treatment

Blood Pressure Control	• Tight control of systolic and diastolic hypertension
Rate Control	• Ventricular rate control for patients with atrial fibrillation to allow for longer filling periods
Diuretics	• Used to control pulmonary edema
Coronary Revascularization	• Consider in patients with known coronary artery disease who remain symptomatic because myocardial ischemia can impair ventricular relaxation
Exercise training	• Should be considered for all stable outpatients with chronic HF who are able to participate in the protocols needed to produce physical conditioning. • Exercise training should be used in conjunction with drug therapy.

3.10.13 Right Ventricular Failure

Signs and Symptoms	Other Features

• Peripheral edema
• Hepatic congestion
• Ascites
• Jugular venous distention
• Right ventricular lift
• Accentuated pulmonic closure sound
• Tricuspid insufficiency murmur
• Pulmonic insufficiency murmur
	• Often accompanies left ventricular failure
	• Associated with primary pulmonary hypertension or secondary pulmonary hypertension caused by conditions such as:
	  - Chronic pulmonary emboli
	  - Sleep-disordered breathing
	  - Interstitial lung disease

Treatment

• Symptomatic treatment with diuretics	• Treat underlying cause

3.10.14 Pharmacologic Therapy

Drug	Starting Dose	Target Dose	Notes
β-Blockers*			
Metoprolol succinate	12.5–25 mg qd depending on BP and HR	200 mg qd	Titrate starting dose up after 2–4 weeks, doubling dose each time until target dose is reached.
Carvedilol	3.125 mg bid	25–50 mg bid	
ACE Inhibitors*			
Captopril	6.25 mg tid	50–100 mg tid	Titrate up after 2–4 weeks until target dose is reached; monitor renal function and electrolytes.
Enalapril	2.5 mg bid	10–20 mg bid	
Ramipril	2.5 mg qd	5 mg bid	
Lisinopril	2.5 mg qd	20–40 mg qd	
Angiotensin II-Receptor Blockers (ARBs)[1]			
Candesartan	4 mg qd	32 mg qd	Titrate up after 2–4 weeks until target dose is reached; monitor renal function and electrolytes.
Valsartan	40 mg bid	160 mg bid	
Aldosterone Antagonists[2]			
Spironolactone	25 mg qd	50 mg qd	Use in addition to β-Blockers and ACEIs once optimal doses have been achieved; titrate up after 2–4 weeks until target dose is reached; monitor renal function and electrolytes
Eplerenone[3]	25 mg qd	50 mg qd	
Other			
Digoxin	0.125 mg qd Monitor renal function; may need to ↓ dose in elderly and renal impairment	0.125–0.25 mg qd	Shown to ↓ hospital admissions, but has no effect on mortality; use in addition to β-blocker, ACEI/ARB, or aldosterone antagonist once optimal doses are achieved
Hydralazine	37.5 mg tid Titrate up after 2–4 weeks until target dose is reached	75 mg tid	Use in combination with isosorbide dinitrate in patients who cannot tolerate ACEI/ARB or in addition to ACEI if aldosterone antagonist is not tolerated; combination shown to ↓ mortality in African Americans

| Isosorbide dinitrate | 20 mg tid Titrate up after 2–4 weeks until target dose is reached | 40 mg tid | Use in combination with hydralazine in patients who cannot tolerate ACEI/ARB or in addition to ACEI if aldosterone antagonist is not tolerated; combination shown to decrease mortality in African Americans. |

*Both β-blockers and ACEIs have been shown to reduce and even reverse LV remodeling and to decrease morbidity and mortality in HF. These drugs are the mainstays of medical management and should be titrated to maximal tolerated doses. [1]ARBs should be substituted for ACEIs in ACEI-intolerant patients. [2]The use of an aldosterone antagonist in combination with an ACEI/ARB or in patients with renal insufficiency can cause life-threatening hyperkalemia and worsening of renal function; electrolytes should be monitored closely. [3]Use in post-MI patients with ejection fraction $\leq$ 40%, heart failure symptoms, or diabetes mellitus.

Diuretic	Initial Dose	Usual Daily Dose
Loop Diuretics		
Furosemide	PO: 20–40 mg qd IV: 10 mg/h	PO: 40–240 mg/d div bid IV: 10–20 mg/h
Bumetanide	PO: 0.5–1 mg qd; IV: 0.5–1 mg/h	PO: 2.5 mg bid; IV: 2–5 mg/h
Torsemide	10–20 mg qd	200 mg/d div bid
Thiazides		
Hydrochlorothiazide	25 mg qd	50 mg qd
Metolazone	2.5 mg qd	2.5–10 mg qd
Natriuretic Peptides		
Nesiritide[4]	2 µg/kg IV bolus, then 0.01 µg/kg/min	0.01–0.03 µg/kg/min

Inotrope	Dosage	Receptor Interaction
Dobutamine	Init 0.5 µg/kg/min, titrate up as needed (max 20 µg/kg/min)	β_1-Agonist
Dopamine	Init 0.5 µg/kg/min, titrate up as needed	3–5 µg/kg/min: β_1-Agonist >10 µg/kg/min: α_1-Agonist
Milrinone	50 µg/kg IV bolus, then 0.375 µg/kg/min; titrate up as needed (max 0.75 µg/kg/min)	cAMP phosphodiesterase inhibitor

Vasodilator	Dose	Adverse Reactions
Nitroglycerine	Init 5–10 µg/kg/min, titrate up as needed (max 200 µg/kg/min)	Tachyphylaxis, hypotension
Nitroprusside	Init 0.25 µg/kg/min, titrate up as needed (max 5 µg/kg/min)	Cyanide toxicity, hypotension

[4]Nesiritide also has vasodilating properties with adverse effects that include hypotension and renal dysfunction; its use is controversial because of conflicting studies on its effect on renal function.

4   Preoperative Evaluation
Prior to Noncardiac Surgery

4.1   Background

- Prevalence of cardiovascular disease is increasing
- Number of non-cardiac surgical procedures performed is increasing
- Preoperative risk assessment is an important step in reducing perioperative morbidity and mortality
- Few basic questions regarding general health, functional capacity, cardiac risk factors, comorbid conditions, and type of operation can assist in evaluating risk
- Not every patient needs a noninvasive test
- A good history and physical examination is very important
- Coronary intervention usually is not necessary to lower the risk of non-cardiac surgery
- Good communication between physicians, anesthesiologists, and surgeons is crucial to minimize risk

4.1.1   Objective

- Purpose of preoperative evaluation is not to clear patients for surgery
- **Note:** Purpose is to assess medical status, cardiac risks posed by the surgery planned, and recommend strategies to reduce risk

4.1.2   Clinical Presentation

- Identify cardiac conditions such as recent MI, decompensated HF, unstable angina, significant arrhythmias, valvular heart disease
- Identify serious comorbid conditions such as diabetes, peripheral vascular disease, stroke, renal insufficiency, pulmonary disease
- Patients with severe aortic stenosis murmur, elevated jugular venous pressure, pulmonary edema, third heart sound have a high surgical risk
- **Assessment of functional capacity**
- **Physical examination**
- **Clinical predictors of risk**

4.1.3 Assessment of Functional Capacity

1 MET	4 METs	< 10 METs
• Eat, dress, use the toilet • Walk indoors around the house • Walk on level ground at 2 mph (3.2 km/h) • Light housework such as washing dishes	• Climb a flight of stairs • Walk on level ground at 4 mph (6.4 km/h) • Run short distance • Vacuuming or lifting heavy furniture • Play golf or doubles tennis	• Swimming • Singles tennis • Basketball • Skiing

MET = metabolic equivalent

4.1.4 Physical Examination

- Blood pressure in both arms
- Carotid pulse
- Jugular venous pressure
- Cardiac rhythm
- Heart sounds (murmurs, gallops)
- Extremity pulses
- Bruits
- Lower extremity edema
- Lung fields
- Abdomen examination for aneurysm
- Ankle-Brachial Index

4.1.5 Clinical Predictors of Risk

Major predictors	Intermediate predictors	Minor predictors
• Recent myocardial infarction with evidence of ischemia based on symptoms or noninvasive testing • Unstable or severe angina • Decompensated CHF • High-grade atrioventricular block • Symptomatic ventricular arrhythmias • Supraventricular arrhythmias with uncontrolled ventricular rate • Severe valvular heart disease	• Mild angina pectoris (Canadian Cardiovascular Class I or II) • Prior MI • Compensated or prior CHF • Diabetes mellitus • Renal insufficiency (Creatinine 2.0 mg/dL)	• Age > 70 y • Abnormal ECG (left ventricular hypertrophy, left bundle branch block, ST-T abnormalities) • Rhythm other than sinus (e.g., atrial fibrillation) • Poor functional capacity • History of stroke • Uncontrolled systemic hypertension

4.1.6   Type of Non-Cardiac Surgery

High-risk surgery	Intermediate-risk surgery	Low-risk surgery
• Emergency major operations, particularly in the elderly • Aortic or peripheral vascular surgery • Extensive operations with large volume shifts	• Intraperitoneal or intrathoracic • Carotid endarterectomy • Head and neck surgery • Orthopedic • Prostate	• Endoscopic procedures • Superficial biopsy • Cataract • Breast surgery

4.1.7   Criteria for Estimating the Risk

Goldman Criteria

Nine variables that independently predict perioperative risk with point value assigned to them in a general surgical population

Age > 70 y	5 points
MI in previous 6 months	10 points
S_3 gallop or jugular venous distention	11 points
Valvular aortic stenosis	3 points
Non sinus rhythm or premature atrial beats	7 points
> 5 premature ventricular beatsper minute	7 points
PO_2 < 60 mm Hg, PCO_2 > 50 mm Hg, K^+ < 3.0 mEq/L or 3.0 mmol/L, HCO_3 < 20 mEq/L or mmol/L, BUN > 50 mg/dL or 18 mmol/L, or Cr > 3.0 mg/dL or 265 mol/L, abnormal AST, chronic liver disease, bedridden patient	3 points
Intraperitoneal, intrathoracic, or aortic operation	3 points
Emergency operation	4 points

Detsky Criteria

Modification of the Goldman criteria to address the severity of coronary artery disease and heart failure in a general surgical population

MI within 6 months	10 points
MI > 6 months prior	5 points
Canadian Cardiovascular Class III angina	10 points
Canadian Cardiovascular Class IV angina	20 points
Unstable angina within 3 months	10 points
Pulmonary edema within 1 week	10 points

Any history of pulmonary edema	5 points
Critical aortic stenosis	20 points
Non-sinus rhythm or atrial premature beats	5 points
> 5 premature ventricular beats at any time	5 points
Poor general medical condition	5 points
Age > 70 y	5 points
Emergency operation	10 points

Eagle Criteria

Uses clinical markers and perfusion imaging in vascular surgery or other major risk category (major thoracic/abdominal surgery)

- Age > 70 y
- Q waves on an ECG
- Diabetes mellitus
- Ventricular arrhythmias necessitating treatment
- History of angina or CHF

≥ 3 risk factors	50% frequency of complications
1–3 risk factors with abnormal thallium	30% frequency of complications
1–3 risk factors with normal thallium	3.2% frequency of complications
0 risk factors	3.1% frequency of complications

Lee Criteria

Six variables that independently predict perioperative risk in a general surgical population

- High-risk surgery
- Ischemic heart disease
- History of CHF
- History of cerebrovascular disease
- Insulin therapy for diabetes
- Serum creatinine ≥ 2.0 mg/dL

Cardiac risk is related to number of risk factors	
0 risk factors	0.4% frequency of complications
1 risk factor	0.9% frequency of complications
2 risk factors	7% frequency of complications
≥ 3 risk factors	11% frequency of complications

4.2 Diagnostic Testing

4.2.1 General Information

- Good history and physical examination are very important
- Laboratory tests
- Noninvasive testing may be indicated in intermediate risk patients
  - Exercise ECG testing
  - Echocardiogram
  - Perfusion imaging and stress echocardiography
- Coronary angiography is only indicated in high risk patients who merit this procedure irrespective of pending noncardiac surgery

4.2.2 Laboratory Testing

- Routine laboratory tests such as creatinine, hemoglobin, platelets, potassium, liver profile, oxygen saturation may be important in risk stratification
- Arterial blood gas is indicated in patients with severe pulmonary disease
- ECG provides important prognostic information
- Patient who are at low risk based on history, physical examination and routine laboratory tests need no further evaluation

4.2.3 Exercise ECG Testing

- Exercise ECG is the modality of choice when noninvasive testing is indicated and patient can walk.
- Exercise ECG provides an estimate of functional capacity, detects myocardial ischemia, and assesses hemodynamic performance during stress.
- Risk stratification based on exercise ECG
- Ability to exercise moderately (4–5 METs) without symptoms defines low risk
- Patients who can achieve > 75% of maximum predicted heart rate without ECG changes are at lowest risk
- Patients with abnormal ECG response at greater than 75% of predicted heart rate are at intermediate risk
- Patients with abnormal ECG response at less than 75% of predicted heart rate are at highest risk
- Perfusion imaging/echocardiogram indicated in patients with abnormal baseline ECG (e.g., LV hypertrophy, digitalis effect)

4.2.4   Echocardiogram

- In patients with a history or signs of HF, preoperative assessment of LV function may be recommended to quantify the severity of systolic and diastolic dysfunction.
- If previous evaluation has documented severe LV dysfunction, repeat preoperative testing may not be necessary.
- Evaluation of a murmur in a patient with cardiorespiratory symptoms or in an asymptomatic patient if the clinical features indicate at least a moderate probability that the murmur is reflective of structural heart disease
- Routine re-evaluation of asymptomatic patients with mild to moderate aortic or mitral stenosis and stable physical signs is not indicated.

4.2.5   Perfusion Nuclear Imaging and Stress Echocardiography

- Stress perfusion imaging indicated in patients with abnormal baseline ECG (e.g., LV hypertrophy, digitalis effect, left bundle branch block)
- Pharmacological perfusion imaging indicated in patients undergoing orthopedic, neurosurgical, or vascular surgery and are unable to exercise, have left bundle branch block, or are paced
- Dipyridamole is contraindicated in patients on theophylline, patients with severe obstructive lung disease, and critical carotid stenosis
- Risk stratification based on perfusion nuclear imaging
- > 4 myocardial segments of redistribution indicates significant risk for perioperative events
- Redistribution in three coronary artery territories indicates higher risk of events.
- Reversible LV cavity dilatation also indicates high risk.
- Total area of ischemia is more predictive than severity of ischemia in a given segment
- Dobutamine stress echocardiography is comparable to dipyridamole thallium testing as a preoperative evaluation tool.
- Dobutamine stress echocardiography is best avoided in patients with severe hypertension, significant arrhythmias, or poor echocardiographic images.

4.2.6 Coronary Angiography Indications

- Indications for coronary angiography before noncardiac surgery are the same as indications for angiography in general (yes, patients should not have angiography just to tide them over for non-cardiac surgery)
- Angina pectoris unresponsive to medical therapy or unstable angina
- High-risk status based on noninvasive testing
- Nondiagnostic noninvasive testing for high-risk patients undergoing high-risk surgery
- Urgent noncardiac surgery on a patient recovering from acute MI
- Current evidence suggests that coronary revascularization before noncardiac surgery is of no value in preventing perioperative cardiac events, except in those patients in whom revascularization is independently indicated for an acute coronary syndrome.

4.3 Therapy

4.3.1 Critical Aortic Stenosis

- Should be recognized preoperatively
- If symptomatic, managed with valve replacement prior to elective surgery
- Valvuloplasty may be considered in selected patients prior to noncardiac surgery in patients with severe aortic stenosis undergoing urgent non-cardiac surgery for a life threatening condition.
- Appropriate prophylaxis for bacterial endocarditis indicated
- Percutaneous aortic valve replacement is being evaluated in several clinical trials and may be an option in the future

4.3.2 Mitral Stenosis

- Medically managed with heart rate control and diuretics when mild and asymptomatic
- If severe or symptomatic, mitral valvuloplasty or surgery may be indicated prior to elective high risk surgery
- Appropriate prophylaxis for bacterial endocarditis indicated

4.3.3 Aortic / Mitral Regurgitation

- Regurgitation lesions are better hemodynamically tolerated than stenotic lesions during surgery
- Medical regimen optimized with diuretics and afterload reduction
- Appropriate prophylaxis for bacterial endocarditis may be indicated

4.3.4 Prosthetic Valves

- Antithrombotic therapy
- Appropriate prophylaxis for bacterial endocarditis indicated

4.3.5 Antithrombotic Therapy

- Usual approach for low risk patients
  - Stop oral anticoagulation 72 hours prior to procedure
  - Restart in the afternoon of day of procedure or after control of active bleeding
- High-risk for thromboembolism (recent thromboembolism, Bjork-Shiley valve, any mechanical valve in mitral position, atrial fibrillation, LV dysfunction):
  - Stop oral anticoagulation 72 hours prior to procedure
  - Start heparin when INR ≤ 2.0
  - Stop heparin 6 hours prior to procedure
  - Restart heparin within 24 hours after procedure and continue until INR ≥ 2.0
- Very low risk surgery (skin surgery, teeth cleaning, caries treatment)
  - Continue antithrombotic therapy

4.3.6 Arrhythmias

- Metabolic profile and medications reviewed and corrected
- Correct even mild hypokalemia
- Sustained or symptomatic ventricular arrhythmias treated with suppressive therapy (i.e., amiodarone) is ok.
- Symptomatic bradyarrhythmias treated with temporary pacing and permanent pacemaker implanted when indicated
- Permanent pacemakers should be checked prior to surgery
- Electrocautery should be minimized in patients who are totally pacemaker-dependent (if extensive electrocautery needed, temporary pacer wire may be considered, with the generator placed as far away as possible from the electrocautery site); magnet only resets the system
- Pacemakers checked after surgery to ensure settings are optimal
- Implanted defibrillators are turned off during surgery and turned back on after surgery

4.3.7 Hypertension

- Mild to moderate hypertensive patients continued on medical therapy and closely monitored during surgery
- Severe hypertension (diastolic BP > 110 mm Hg) need optimization of therapy and adequate control prior to surgery
- For urgent surgery in patients with severe hypertension, intravenous agents are used
- Withdrawal of β-Blockers and clonidine should be avoided

4.3.8 Cardiomyopathy

- Pulmonary artery catheter sometimes may benefit patients with severe LV dysfunction but not routinely recommended
- Close monitoring of volume status, heart rate, and systemic vascular resistance in hypertrophic cardiomyopathy

4.3.9 Coronary Artery Disease

- Noncardiac surgery does not alter the indications for revascularization
- Perioperative use of β-Blockers is beneficial in selected patients
- Nitroglycerin indicated for high risk patients
- Current guidelines state that for patients currently taking statins and scheduled for noncardiac surgery, statins should be continued; for patients undergoing vascular surgery with or without clinical risk factors, statin use is reasonable
- Antiplatelet agents such as aspirin, which may have been temporarily discontinued prior to surgery, should be reinitiated when no longer contraindicated.

4.3.10 Beta Blockers

- β-Blockers reduce myocardial oxygen demand
- β-Blockers reduce myocardial oxygen consumption by suppressing lipolysis
- The ACC/AHA 2009 Guideline Update on Perioperative Cardiovascular Evaluation for Noncardiac Surgery: Focused Update on Perioperative β-Blocker Therapy recommends as a Class I indication that β-Blockers should be continued in patients undergoing surgery who are receiving β-Blockers to treat angina, symptomatic arrhythmias, hypertension, or other current ACC/AHA Class I guideline indications
- On the other hand, routine administration of high-dose β-Blockers in the absence of dose titration is not useful and may be harmful to patients not currently taking beta blockers who are undergoing noncardiac surgery

4.3.11 Carotid Stenosis

- Significant cardiac events reported in patients with carotid stenosis and abnormal thallium scans
- Treatment strategy for patients with significant coronary artery disease and carotid stenosis is controversial
- Combined carotid endarterectomy and CABG reserved for patients with severe neurological symptoms and unstable angina

4.3.12 Perioperative Management

- Mortality rate as high as 50% with perioperative MI
- For patients with coronary disease, monitor ECG and cardiac enzymes after surgery
- Pulmonary artery catheters may be beneficial for patients with severe LV dysfunction at risk for HF

4.3.13 Postoperative Management

- Postoperative cardiac evaluation indicated for patients who underwent urgent surgery or who did not have preoperative evaluation
- Management of risk factors such as hypertension, diabetes, hyperlipidemia important
- Aggressive treatment including revascularization indicated for patients with perioperative MI or ischemia

4.3.14 General Recommendations

- It is important to determine the urgency of noncardiac surgery. In many cases patient- or surgery-specific factors dictate immediate surgery and may not allow further cardiac assessment or treatment.
- Patients who have a need for emergency noncardiac surgery should proceed to the operating room and continue perioperative surveillance and postoperative risk stratification and risk factor management.
- Patients with active cardiac conditions should be evaluated and treated per ACC/AHA guidelines and, if appropriate, consider proceeding to the operating room.
- Patients undergoing low-risk surgery are recommended to proceed to planned surgery.
- Patients with poor (less than 4 METs) or unknown functional capacity and no clinical risk factors should proceed with planned surgery
- It is probably recommended that patients with poor (less than 4 METs) or unknown functional capacity and 3 or more clinical risk factors, who are scheduled for vascular surgery, consider testing if it will change management.
- It is probably recommended that patients with functional capacity greater than or equal to 4 METs without symptoms proceed to planned surgery.

4.3.15 Cardiac Evaluation and Care Algorithm for Noncardiac Surgery

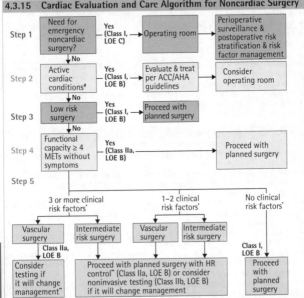

Cardiac Evaluation and Care Algorithm for Noncardiac Surgery Based on Active Clinical Conditions, Known Cardiovascular Disease, or Cardiac Risk for Patients 50 Years of Age or Greater. # Active cardiac conditions include unstable coronary syndromes, decompensated HF (NYHA functional class IV; worsening or new-onset HF), significant arrhythmias and severe valvular heart disease. * Clinical risk factors include ischemic heart disease, compensated or prior heart failure, diabetes mellitus, renal insufficiency, and cerebrovascular disease. ** Consider perioperative β-Blockade for populations in which this has been shown to reduce cardiac morbidity/mortality. Reprinted from the Journal of the American College of Cardiology, 50 (17), Fleisher LA, et al. ACC/AHA 2007 Guidelines on Perioperative Cardiovascular Evaluation and Care for Noncardiac Surgery: Executive Summary, 1707–1732. Copyright 2007, with permission from the American College of Cardiology Foundation and the American Heart Association, Inc. Published by Elsevier Inc.

5 Cardiovascular Drugs

5.1 Vasopressors (See abbreviations inside the cover)

MA/EF (dobutamine): primarily β-receptor agonist, pos. inotropic, no vasoconstriction;
MA/EF (dopamine): dose-dependent dopamine-, β-/α-receptor agonist; renal vasodilation (D_1-mediated), cardiac output ↑ ($β_1$-mediated pos. ino- and chronotropic), in high doses cardiac output ↓ ($α_1$-vasoconstriction ⇒ heart rate ↓)
MA/EF (epinephrine): primarily β-receptor agonist, pos. inotropic, chronotropic + bathmotropic effect, systolic BP ↑, diastolic BP ↓, bronchodilation
MA/EF (norepinephrine): primarily α-receptor agonist ⇒ syst./diast. BP ↑
MA/EF (midodrine): α-adrenergic agonism on arteriolar + venous receptors ⇒ vascular tone ↑, venous pooling ↓, BP ↑
MA/EF (metaraminol) release of norepinephrine + direct α-(β-1) receptor agonism⇒ vasoconstriction, BP ↑
MA/EF (methoxamine): α-1 sel. rec. agon. ⇒ periph. resistance ↑, BP ↑ ⇒ sinus bradycardia
AE: headache, anxiety, fatigue, N/V, dyspnea, angina, hypertension/hypotension, arrhythmias, parasthesia, bradycardia, palpitations, hyperglycemia
CI: thyrotoxicosis, pheochromocytoma, glaucoma, difficult urination, tachyarrhythmia, acute MI, aortic valve stenosis, hypertension, combination with systemic β-2 sympathomimetics;
CI (dobutamine): pheochromocytoma, idiopathic hypertrophic subaortic stenosis, drug hypersensitivity;
CI (dopamine): pheochromocytoma;
CI (epinephrine) narrow angle glaucoma, anesthesia with halogenated hydrocarbons/cyclopropane, organic brain damage, labor, cardiac dilatation, coronary insuffic.
CI (norepinephrine): anesthesia with halogenated hydrocarbons/cyclopropane, vascular thrombosis;
CI (midodrine): excessive supine hypertension, severe organic heart disease, acute renal disease, urinary retention, pheochromocytoma, thyrotoxicosis, drug hypersensitivity;
CI (methoxamine): drug hypersensitivity, severe HTN, local anesthetics

Dobutamine	
	EHL 2min, Dur (1x dose) 10min, Q0 0.7, PRC B, Lact ?
Generics Inj 12.5mg/ml, 50mg/100ml, 100mg/100ml, 200mg/100ml, 400mg/100ml, 1.25g/100ml	Cardiac decompensation: ini 0.5-1µg/kg/min IV, incr to 2-20µg/kg/min, max 40µg/kg/min

Dopamine	
	EHL 2min, Dur 10min, Q0 0.95, PRC C, Lact ?
Generics Inj 1.6mg/ml, 40mg/ml, 80mg/ml, 160mg/ml, 80mg/100ml, 160mg/100ml, 320mg/100ml, 640mg/100ml	Hypotension, heart failure: ini 1-5µg/kg/min IV, incr prn by 5-10µg/kg/min increments, max 50µg/kg/min;

Ephedrine sulfate	
	EHL 3h, PRC C, Lact ?
Generics Inj 50mg/ml	Acute hypotension: 25-50mg SC/IM; CH: 750µg/kg IV/SC

Epinephrine	EHL 1min, Q0 >0.7, PRC C, Lact ?
Adrenaclick *Inj (IM/SC) 0.15, 0.3mg/delivery* **Epipen Jr.** *Inj (IM) 0.15mg/delivery* **Epipen** *Inj (IM) 0.3mg/delivery* **Twinject** *Inj (IM/SC) 0.15, 0.3mg/delivery* **Generics** *Inj (IM) 0.15mg/delivery*	**Cardiac arrest:** 0.5-1mg IV/ET, rep prn q3-5min; anaphylaxis: 0.3-0.5 mg SC/IM, rep prn q10-15min; **CH:** 0.01mg/kg IV; 0.1mg/kg ET rep prn with 0.1mg/kg IV/ET q3-5min; **anaphylaxis:** 0.01mg/kg SC/IM (use 1: 1000 Sol), then 0.1mg/kg IV prn (IV: use 1:10,000)

Metaraminol	Dur 20-60min, PRC C, Lact ?
Generics *Inj 10mg/ml*	**Acute hypotension (in surgery, spinal anesthesia):** 0.5-5mg IV, then inf of 15-100mg in 500ml; 2-10mg SC; DARF: not req

Midodrine	EHL 0.5h, Q0 0.4, PRC C, Lact ?
ProAmatine *Tab 2.5mg, 5mg, 10mg* **Orvaten** *Tab 2.5mg, 5mg, 10mg* **Generics** *Tab 2.5mg, 5mg, 10mg*	**Orthostatic hypotension:** ini 10mg PO tid, incr prn to max 40mg/d; DARF: ini 2.5mg tid

Norepinephrine	Dur 1-2min, Q0 >0.8, PRC C, Lact ?
Levophed *Inj 1mg/ml* **Generics** *Inj 1mg/ml*	**Acute hypotensive states:** ini 8-12 µg/min IV, maint 2-4 µg/min

Phenylephrine	PRC C, Lact ?
Neo-Synephrine *Inj 10mg/ml* **Generics** *Inj 10mg/ml*	**Acute hypotension:** 2-5mg SC/IM, max ini 5mg IV, rep prn q1-2h; 0.2-0.5mg slowly IV, max ini 0.5mg IV

5.2 Beta Blockers

MA: competitive blockage of β-receptors; **EF:** neg. inotropic + chronotropic ⇒ cardiac output ↓, myocardial O_2 consumption ↓, renin secret. ↓, high-dose nonspecif. membrane-stabilizing effect (quinidine-like); **AE:** avoid in decompensated heart failure until stabilized; (acebutalol): bradycardia, bronchospasm, fatigue, dyspnea, nausea, dizziness, hypotens., rash; **AE** (atenolol): AV block, bradycardia, bronchospasm, dizziness, vertigo, fatigue, diarrhea, nausea, dry mouth; **AE** (bisoprolol): arthralgia, dizziness, headache, insomnia, diarrhea, nausea, coughing, fatigue, edema; **AE** (carvedilol): syncope, bradycardia, hypotension, fatigue, dizziness, dyspnea; **AE** (esmolol): hypotens., bradycardia, bronchospasm; **AE** (labetalol): hypotension, jaundice, bronchospasm, dizziness, fatigue, headache, angina, nausea; **AE** (metoprolol/nadolol): hypotension, bradycardia, AV block, bradycardia, hypotension, peripheral vasoconstriction, bronchospasm, N/V, constipat., diarrhea, sexual ability ↓, insulin secretion ↓, glycogenolysis ↓, fatigue, insomnia, dizziness, drowsiness, weakness, nervousness, anxiety, mental depression; **AE** (propranolol): bronchospasm, anorexia, N/V, diarrhea, abdominal pain; **CI** (betablockers): bronchospasm, sinus bradycardia, second and third degree AV block, RV failure, secondary pulmonary hypertension, cardiogenic shock, hypersensitivity to drug; **CI** (acebutalol/bisoprolol): anesthesia that produces cardiac depression; **CI** (atenolol): sick sinus syndrome, severe PVD, pheochromocytoma without α-blockade, metabolic acidosis; **CI** (carvedilol): severe hypotension, hepatic impairment, mental incapacity; **CI** (metoprolol): severe PVD, anesthesia producing cardiac depression; **CI** (nadolol): allergic rhinitis; **CI** (pindolol): anesthesia producing cardiac depression; **CI** (propranolol): allergic rhinitis

		β_1	ISA
Acebutolol	EHL 3-4h, Q0 0.8 (0.4), PRC B, Lact ?	+	+
Sectral *Cap 200mg, 400mg* **Generics** *Cap 200mg, 400mg*	**HTN:** ini 400mg PO qd or 200mg PO bid, maint 400-800mg/d, max 1200mg/d; **ventricular arrhythmia:** ini 200mg PO bid, maint 0.6-1.2g/d; DARF: GFR (ml/min) 25-50: 50%; <25: 25%		
Atenolol	EHL 6-7h, Q0 0.12, PRC D, Lact ?	+	-
Tenormin *Tab 25mg, 50mg,* **Generics** *Tab 25mg, 50mg,* *100mg*	**Post MI:** 100mg PO qd or div bid; **HTN:** ini 50mg PO qd, maint 50-100mg/d; **angina:** 50-200mg PO qd; DARF: GFR (ml/min) 15-35: max 50mg/d PO/IV; <15: max 25mg/d PO or 50mg/d IV		
Betaxolol	EHL 12-22h, Q0 0.8, PRC C, Lact ?	+	-
Kerlone *Tab 10, 20mg* **Generics** *Tab 10, 20mg*	**HTN:** ini 10mg PO qd, max 20mg/d; DARF: ini 5mg PO, incr by 5mg q14d, max 20mg/d		
Bisoprolol	EHL 10-12.4h, Q0 0.48, PRC C, Lact ?	+	-
Zebeta *Tab 5mg, 10mg* **Generics** *Tab 5mg, 10mg*	**HTN:** 2.5-5mg PO qd, max 20mg/d; DARF: ini 2.5mg PO qd, incr prn		
Carvedilol	EHL 6-10h, Q0 1.0, PRC C, Lact ?	-	-
Coreg *Tab 3.125mg, 6.25mg,* *12.5mg, 25mg;* *Tab ext. rel. 10mg, 20mg,* *40mg, 80mg*	**Heart failure:** ini 3.125mg PO bid or 10mg qd, incr dose q2 wk as tolerated to max 25mg bid (<85 kg) or 50mg bid (>85 kg) or 80mg qd; **HTN:** ini 6.25mg PO bid or 20mg qd, incr prn, max 80mg/d; DARF: not req		
Esmolol	EHL 9min, Q0 1.0, PRC C, Lact ?	+	-
Brevibloc *Inj 10mg/ml, 20mg/* *ml, 250mg/ml,* *1g/100ml, 2g/100ml* **Generics** *10mg/ml*	**SV tachyarrhythmia:** 500µg/kg IV over 1min, then 50µg/kg/min IV over 4min; DARF: not req		
Labetalol	EHL 5-8h, PRC C, Lact +	-	(+)
Trandate *Tab 100mg, 200mg,* *300mg, Inj 5mg/ml* **Generics** *Tab 100mg, 200mg,* *300mg, Inj 5mg/ml*	**Hypertensive emergency:** 20mg slow IV, then 40-80mg IV q10min prn, max 300mg total; **HTN:** ini 100mg PO bid, maint 200-400mg bid, max 2400mg/d; DARF: not req		
Metoprolol	EHL 3-7h, PRC C, Lact ?	+	-
Lopressor *Tab 50mg, 100mg,* *Inj 1mg/ml* **Toprol-xl** *Tab ext.rel 25mg,* *50mg, 100mg, 200mg* **Generics** *Tab 50mg, 100mg,* *Inj 1mg/ml*	**HTN, angina:** ini 50mg PO bid or 50-100mg PO qd (ext.rel), incr prn max 400mg/d; **acute MI:** ini 5mg IV q2min up to 15mg, if tolerated give 50mg PO q6h for 48h, then 100mg PO bid; **heart failure:** ini 6.25-12.5mg PO bid, incr q2 wk as tolerated max 200mg/d; DARF: not req		
Nadolol	EHL 20-24h, Q0 0.4, PRC C, Lact ?	+	-
Corgard *Tab 20mg, 40mg,* *80mg* **Generics** *Tab 20mg, 40mg,* *80mg*	**HTN:** ini 40mg PO qd, maint 40-80mg/d, max 320mg/d; **angina:** ini 40mg PO qd, maint 40-80mg/d, max 240mg/d; DARF: GFR (ml/min): >50: q24h, 31-50: q24-36h, 10-30: q24-48h, <10: q40-60h		

			β_1	ISA
Nebivolol		EHL 12-19h, Q0 0.95, PRC C, Lact ?		
Bystolic *Tab 2.5mg, 5mg, 10mg, 20mg*	**HTN:** ini 5mg PO qd, incr prn at 2wk intervals to max 40mg/d; DARF: GFR (ml/min) <30: ini 2.5mg		+	–
Penbutolol		EHL 17-26h, Q0 0.95, PRC C, Lact ?	–	+
Levatol *Tab 20mg*	**Angina pectoris:** 10-40mg PO qd; **HTN:** 20mg PO qd; DARF: not req			
Pindolol		EHL 3-4h, Q0 0.5, PRC B, Lact ?	–	+
Generics *Tab 5mg, 10mg*	**Angina pectoris:** ini 2.5-5mg/d PO, maint 10-40mg/d div tid; **HTN:** ini 5mg PO bid, maint 10-40mg/d, max 60mg/d; DARF: not req			
Propranolol		EHL 3-4h, Q0 1.0, PRC C, Lact ?	–	–
Inderal *Tab 10mg, 20mg, 40mg, 60mg, 80mg, Inj 1mg/ml* **Inderal LA** *Cap ext.rel 60mg, 80mg, 120mg, 160mg* **Innopran XL** *Cap ext.rel 80mg, 120mg* **Generics** *Tab 10mg, 20mg, 40mg, 60mg, 80mg, 90mg, Sol (oral) 20mg/5ml, 40mg/5ml, 80mg/ml, Inj 1mg/ml*	**HTN:** ini 40mg PO bid, maint 120-240mg/d, max 640mg/d; ext.rel: ini 60-80mg PO qd, maint 120-160mg/d, max 640mg/d; **angina:** ini 10-20mg PO tid-qid, maint 160-240mg/d; **arrhythmias:** 1-3mg IV, rep after 2min prn; 10-30mg PO tid-qid; **MI:** 180-240mg/d PO div bid-qid; **migraine:** ini 80 mg/d PO, maint 160-240mg/d; **essential tremor:** ini 40mg/d PO, maint 120mg/d; **pheochromocytoma:** preop. 60mg/d PO in div doses bid-tid in combination with an α- blocking agent; **hypertrophic subaortic stenosis:** 20-40mg PO bid-tid; **CH** 2-4mg/kg/d PO div bid; DARF: not req			
Timolol		EHL 2-4h, PRC C, Lact ?	–	–
Generics *Tab 5mg, 10mg, 20mg*	**HTN:** ini 10mg PO bid, maint 20-40mg/d, max 60mg/d; **MI:** 10mg PO bid; **migraine:** ini 10mg PO bid, maint 20mg/d qd; DARF: not req			

β_1: selective blockage of β-1 receptors; **ISA:** intrinsic sympathomimetic activity = partial agonistic and antagonist activity

5.3 ACE Inhibitors

5.3.1 ACE Inhibitors: Single Ingredient Drugs

MA: competitive block. of angiotensin convert. enzyme ⇒ angiotensin II ↓, bradykinin ↑
EF: vasodil. ⇒ BP ↓, renal blood flow↑, aldosterone ↓, catecholamines ↓, reversal of myocard. + blood vessel wall hypertrophy, protect. in diabetic nephrop.;
AE: acute RF, rash, dry cough, hair loss, angioedema, dizziness, fatigue, angioneurotic edema, headache, K+ ↑, Na+ ↓, complete blood count changes, urticaria, hypotension;
CI: angiodema, hypersensitiv. to drug

Benazepril	EHL 0.6 h, Q0 0.05, PRC C(1), D(2nd, 3rd trim.), Lact ↓
Lotensin *Tab 5mg, 10mg, 20mg, 40mg* **Generics** *Tab 5mg, 10mg, 20mg, 40mg*	**HTN:** ini 10mg PO qd, maint 20-40mg PO qd or div bid, max 80mg/d; DARF: GFR (ml/min) >50: 100%; 10-50: 50-75%; <10: 25-50%

Captopril	EHL 1.9h, Q0 0.15, PRC C(1), D(2nd, 3rd trim.), Lact +
Capoten *Tab 12.5mg, 25mg, 50mg, 100mg* **Generics** *Tab 12.5mg, 25mg, 50mg, 100mg*	**HTN**: ini 25mg PO bid-tid, maint 25-150mg PO bid-tid, max 450mg/d; **heart failure**: ini 12.5-25mg PO tid, incr to 150-300mg/d div tid, max 450mg/d; DARF: GFR (ml/min) >50: 100% q8h; 10-50: 50-75% q12-18h; <10: 25-50% q24h
Enalapril	EHL 1.3h, Q0 0.1, PRC C(1st), D(2nd, 3rd trim.), Lact +
Vasotec *Tab 2.5mg, 5mg, 10mg, 20mg* **Generics** *Tab 2.5mg, 5mg, 10mg, 20mg;* *Inj 1.25mg/ml*	**HTN**: ini 5mg PO qd, maint 10-40mg PO qd or div bid, max 40mg/d; 1.25mg IV q6h, max 5mg IV q6h; **heart failure**: ini 2.5 mg PO bid, incr to 10-20mg PO bid, max 40mg/d; **CH heart failure**: 0.1-0.5mg/kg/d PO qd or div bid; DARF: GFR (ml/min) <30: ini 2.5mg PO qd, titrate prn, max 40mg/d
Fosinopril	EHL 11.5h, Q0 0.5, PRC C(1st), D(2nd, 3rd trim.), Lact +
Monopril *Tab 10mg, 20mg, 40mg* **Generics** *Tab 10mg, 20mg, 40mg*	**HTN**: ini 10mg PO qd, maint 10-40mg PO qd, max 80mg/d; **heart failure**: ini 5-10mg PO qd, maint 20-40mg PO qd, max 40mg/d; DARF: not req
Lisinopril	EHL 12h, Q0 0.3, PRC C(1st), D(2nd, 3rd trim.), Lact +
Zestril *Tab 2.5mg, 5mg, 10mg, 20mg, 30mg, 40mg* **Prinivil** *Tab 2.5mg, 5mg, 10mg, 20mg, 40mg* **Generics** *Tab 2.5, mg, 5mg, 10mg, 20mg, 30mg, 40mg*	**HTN**: ini 10mg PO qd, maint 20-40mg PO qd, max 80mg/d; **heart failure**: ini 2.5-5mg PO qd, maint 5-40mg PO qd, max 80mg/d; DARF: GFR (ml/min) 10-30: ini 5mg PO, <10: ini 2.5mg PO, titrate dosage prn, max 40mg/d
Moexipril	EHL 1 h, Q0 (0.4), PRC C(1st), D(2nd, 3rd trim.), Lact +
Univasc *Tab 7.5mg, 15mg* **Generics** *Tab 7.5mg, 15mg*	**HTN**: ini 7.5mg PO qd, maint 7.5-30mg PO qd, max 60mg/d; DARF: GFR (ml/min) <40: 3.75mg PO qd
Perindopril	EHL 0.9 h, Q0 (0.56), PRC C(1st), D(2nd, 3rd trim.), Lact +
Aceon *Tab 2mg, 4mg, 8mg* **Generics** *Tab 2mg, 4mg, 8mg*	**HTN**: ini 4mg PO qd, maint 4-8mg PO qd, max 16mg/d; **stable coronary artery disease**: <70y: ini 4mg PO qd for 2wk, incr as tolerated to 8mg/d; >70y: d1-7 2mg qd, d8-14 4mg qd, then 8mg as tolerated; DARF: GFR (ml/min) <30: ini 2mg PO qd, max 8mg/d
Quinapril	EHL 0.8h, Q0 0.2, PRC C(1st), D(2nd, 3rd trim.), Lact +
Accupril *Tab 5mg, 10mg, 20mg, 40mg* **Generics** *Tab 5mg, 10mg, 20mg, 40mg*	**HTN**: ini 10mg PO qd, maint 20-80mg PO qd or div bid, max 80mg/d; **heart failure**: ini 5mg PO qd-bid, maint 20-40mg/d div bid; DARF: GFR (ml/min) >60: ini 10mg PO; 30-60: ini 5mg PO; 10-30: ini 2.5mg PO, then titrate to the optimal response

Ramipril	EHL 1–5h, Q0 0.15, PRC C(1st), D(2nd, 3rd trim.), Lact +
Altace *Cap 1.25mg, 2.5mg, 5mg, 10mg* **Generics** *Cap 1.25mg, 2.5mg, 5mg, 10mg*	**HTN:** ini 2.5mg PO qd, maint 2.5-20mg PO qd or div bid, max 20mg/d; **heart failure:** ini 1.25-2.5mg PO bid, maint 2.5-5mg bid, max 10mg/d; DARF: GFR (ml/min) < 40: 25%

Trandolapril	EHL 0.6–1.3h, Q0 0.44, PRC C(1), D(2nd,3rd trim.), Lact +
Mavik *Tab 1mg, 2mg, 4mg* **Generics** *Tab 1mg, 2mg, 4mg*	**HTN, heart failure:** ini 1mg PO qd, maint 2-4mg PO qd, max 8mg/d; DARF: GFR (ml/min) <30: ini 0.5mg, titrate to optimal response

5.3.2 ACE Inhibitors: Combinations

Benazepril + Hydrochlorothiazide (HCTZ)	PRC C(1st trim.), D(2nd, 3rd trim.), Lact -
Lotensin HCT *Tab 10 + 12.5mg, 20 + 12.5mg, 20 + 25mg, 5 + 6.25mg* **Generics** *Tab 10 + 12.5mg, 20 + 12.5mg, 5 + 6.25mg*	**HTN:** 5+6.25 - 20+25mg PO qd; DARF: GFR (ml/min) >30: 100%, <30: not rec

Captopril + HCTZ	PRC C(1st trim.), D(2nd, 3rd trim.), Lact -
Capozide *Tab 25 + 15mg, 25 + 25mg, 50 + 15mg, 50 + 25mg* **Generics** *Tab 25 + 15mg, 25 + 25mg, 50 + 15mg, Tab 50 + 25mg*	**HTN:** 25+15 - 50+25mg PO qd-bid; DARF: GFR (ml/min) >30: 100%, <30: not rec

Enalapril + HCTZ	PRC C(1st trim.), D(2nd, 3rd trim.), Lact -
Vaseretic *Tab 5 + 12.5mg, 10 + 25mg* **Generics** *Tab 5 + 12.5mg, 10 + 25mg*	**HTN:** 5+12.5 - 10+25mg PO qd, max 20+50mg PO qd or div bid; DARF: GFR (ml/min) >30: 100%, <30: not rec

Fosinopril + HCTZ	PRC C(1st trim.), D(2nd, 3rd trim.), Lact -
Monopril-HCT *Tab 10 + 12.5mg, 20 + 12.5mg* **Generics** *Tab 10 + 12.5mg, 20 + 12.5mg*	**HTN:** 10+12.5 - 20+12.5mg PO qd; DARF: GFR (ml/min) >30: 100%, <30: not rec

Lisinopril + HCTZ	PRC C(1st trim.), D(2nd, 3rd trim.), Lact -
Prinzide *Tab 10 + 12.5mg, 20 + 12.5mg, 20 + 25mg* **Zestoretic** *Tab 10 + 12.5mg, 20 + 12.5mg, 20 + 25mg* **Generics** *ab 10 + 12.5mg, 20 + 12.5mg, 20 + 25mg*	**HTN:** 10+12.5 - 20+25mg PO qd; DARF: GFR (ml/min) >30: 100%, <30: not rec

Moexipril + HCTZ	PRC C(1st trim.), D(2nd, 3rd trim.), Lact -
Uniretic *Tab 7.5 + 12.5mg; 15 + 12.5mg; 15 + 25mg;*	**HTN:** 7.5+12.5 - 15+25mg PO qd, max 30+50mg PO; GFR (ml/min) >40: 100%, <40: not rec

Quinapril + HCTZ	PRC C(1st trim.), D(2nd, 3rd trim.), Lact -
Accuretic Tab 10 + 12.5mg, 20 + 12.5mg, 20 + 25mg **Quinaretic** Tab 10 + 12.5mg, 20 + 12.5mg, 20 + 25mg **Generics** Tab 10 + 12.5mg, 20 + 12.5mg, 20 + 25mg	**HTN:** 10+12.5 - 20+25mg PO, max 40+25mg PO qd; DARF: GFR (ml/min) >30: 100%, <30: not req

5.4   Angiotensin II Receptor Blockers

5.4.1   Angiotensin II Receptor Blockers: Single Ingredient Drugs

MA (ARBs): inhibition of type 1 angiotensin II receptor
EF: selective blockage of angiotensin II-effects without action on bradykinin breakdown;
AE: headache, dizziness, nausea, abdominal pain;
CI: hypersensitivity to drug

Candesartan	Q0 0.4, PRC C(1st), D(2nd, 3rd trim.), Lact ?
Atacand Tab 4mg, 8mg, 16mg, 32mg	**HTN:** ini 16mg PO qd, max 32mg/d; **heart failure:** (NYHA II-IV): ini 4mg PO qd, double dose if tolerated q2wk to 32mg/d; DARF: not req
Eprosartan	EHL 6h, Q0 0.9, PRC C(1st), D(2nd, 3rd trim.), Lact -
Teveten Tab 400mg, 600mg	**HTN:** ini 600mg PO qd, max 800mg qd
Irbesartan	EHL 11-15h, Q0 1.0, PRC C(1), D(2nd, 3rd trim.), Lact ?
Avapro Tab 75mg, 150mg, 300mg	**HTN:** ini 150mg PO qd, max 300mg/d; **diabetic nephropathy:** 300mg PO qd; DARF: not req
Losartan	EHL 1.5-2h, Q0 0.95, PRC C(1.), D(2nd, 3rd trim.), Lact ?
Cozaar Tab 25mg, 50mg, 100mg **Generics** Tab 25mg, 50mg, 100mg	**HTN:** ini 50mg PO qd, max 100mg qd or div bid; **heart failure:** ini 12.5mg PO qd, incr in 7d intervals to 25-50mg/d; **diabetic nephropathy:** ini 50mg PO qd, then 100mg qd, DARF: not req
Olmesartan	EHL 13h, PRC C(1st), D(2nd, 3rd trim.), Lact ?
Benicar Tab 5mg, 20mg, 40mg	**HTN:** ini 20mg PO qd, incr prn to 40mg qd
Telmisartan	EHL 24h, Q0 1.0, PRC C(1st), D(2nd, 3rd trim.), Lact ?
Micardis Tab 20mg, 40mg, 80mg	**HTN:** ini 40mg PO qd, max 80mg/d
Valsartan	EHL 6-9h, Q0 0.7, PRC C(1st), D(2nd, 3rd trim.), Lact ?
Diovan Cap 40mg, 80mg, 160mg, 320mg	**HTN:** ini 80mg PO qd, max 320mg/d; **heart failure:** ini 40mg PO bid, incr as tolerated to max. 320mg/d in divided doses; **post-MI left ventricular dysfunction:** ini 20mg bid, incr to 40mg bid within 7d, incr as tolerated to 160mg bid; DARF: GFR (ml/min) >10: not req

5.4.2 Angiotensin II Receptor Blockers: Combinations

Candesartan + HCTZ	PRC C(1st), D(2nd, 3rd trim.), Lact -
Atacand HCT Tab 16 + 12.5mg, 32 + 12.5mg, 32 + 25mg	**HTN:** 16+12.5 - 300+12.5mg PO qd; **DARF:** GFR (ml/min) >30: 100%, <30: not rec
Eprosartan + HCTZ	PRC C(1st), D(2nd, 3rd trim.), Lact -
Teveten HCT Tab 600 + 12.5mg, 600 + 25mg	**HTN:** 600+12.5-25mg PO qd; **DARF:** GFR (ml/min) >30: 100%, <30: not rec
Irbesartan + HCTZ	PRC C(1st), D(2nd, 3rd trim.), Lact -
Avalide Tab 150 + 12.5mg, 300 + 12.5mg, 300 + 25mg	**HTN:** 150+12.5 - 300+25mg PO qd **DARF:** GFR (ml/min) >30: 100%, <30: not rec
Losartan + HCTZ	PRC C(1st), D(2nd, 3rd trim.), Lact -
Hyzaar Tab 50 + 12.5mg, 100 + 12.5mg, 100 + 25mg **Generics** Tab 50 + 12.5mg, 100 + 12.5mg, 100 + 25mg	**HTN:** 50+12.5 - 100+25mg PO qd **DARF:** GFR (ml/min) >30: 100%, <30: not rec
Olmesartan + HCTZ	EHL 13h, PRC C(1st), D(2nd, 3rd trim.), Lact -
Benicar HCT Tab 20 + 12.5mg, 40 + 12.5mg, 40 + 25mg	**HTN:** 20+12.5 - 40+25mg PO qd; **DARF:** GFR (ml/min) >30: 100%, <30: not rec
Telmisartan + HCTZ	EHL 24h, PRC C(1st), D(2nd, 3rd trim.), Lact -
Micardis HCT Tab 40 + 12.5mg, 80 + 12.5mg, 80 + 25mg	**HTN:** 40+12.5 - 160+25mg PO qd; **DARF:** GFR (ml/min) >30: 100%, <30: not rec
Valsartan + HCTZ	PRC C(1st), D(2nd, 3rd trim.), Lact -
Diovan HCT Tab 80 + 12.5mg, 160 + 12.5mg, 160 + 25mg, 320 + 12.5mg, 320 + 25mg	**HTN:** 80+12.5 - 320+25mg PO qd **DARF:** GFR (ml/min) >30: 100%, <30: not rec

5.5 Renin Inhibitors

5.5.1 Renin Inhibitors: Single Ingredient Drugs

MA (Aliskiren): direct renin inhibitior ⇒ plasma renin activity ↓ ⇒ inhibition of conversion from angiotensinogen to Angiotensin I ⇒ BP↓; **AE** (Aliskiren): diarrhea, GERD, hyperkalemia, angioedema, severe hypotension; **CI** (Aliskiren): hypersensitiv. to Aliskiren, pregnancy

Aliskiren	EHI 24h PRC C(1st), D(2nd, 3rd trim.), Lact ?
Tekturna Tab 150mg, 300mg	**HTN:** ini 150mg PO qd, incr prn to 300mg qd; **DARF:** caution advised in severe RF

5.5.2 Renin Inhibitors: Combinations

Aliskiren + Amlodipine	PRC D, Lact ?
Tekamlo Tab 150 + 5mg, 150 + 10mg, 300 + 5mg, 300 + 10mg	**HTN:** ini 150+5mg PO qd, incr. prn to max 300+10mg qd; **DARF:** mild-moderate RF: not req.; severe RF: no data
Aliskiren + HCTZ	PRC D, Lact ?
Tekturna HCT Tab 150 + 12.5mg, 150 + 25mg, 300 + 12.5mg, 300 + 25mg	**HTN:** 1 Tab PO qd, incr prn to max 300 + 25mg; **DARF:** GFR (ml/min) <30: not rec

Aliskiren + Valsartan	PRC D, Lact ?
Valturna *Tab 150 + 160mg, 300 + 320mg*	**HTN**: ini 150+160mg PO qd, incr. prn to 300+320mg qd; DARF: no data

5.6 Calcium Channel Blockers

5.6.1 CCBs: Dihydropyridines

MA: blockage of inflow of calcium ions ⇒ neg. inotropic effect, myocardial O_2 consumption ↓, predominantly arterial vasodilation ⇒ afterload ↓, preload unchanged
AE: hypotension, flush, reflex tachycardia, ankle edema, headache, complete blood count changes, gingival hyperplasia;
CI: hypersensitivity to drug, severe hypotension

Amlodipine	EHL 35-50h, Q0 0.85, PRC C, Lact ?
Norvasc *Tab 2.5mg, 5mg, 10mg* **Generics** *Tab 2.5mg, 5mg, 10mg*	**HTN**: ini 2.5-5mg PO qd, max 10mg qd; **chronic stable AP**: 5-10mg PO qd; DARF: not req

Felodipine	EHL 10-16h, Q0 1.0, PRC C, Lact ?
Plendil *Tab ext.rel 10mg, 2.5mg, 5mg* **Generics** *Tab ext.rel 10mg, 2.5mg, 5mg*	**HTN**: ini 5mg PO qd, maint 5-10mg/d; DARF: not req

Isradipine	EHL 5-10.7h, Q0 1.0, PRC C, Lact ?
Dynacirc *Cap 2.5mg* **Dynacirc CR** *Tab ext.rel 5mg, 10mg* **Generics** *Cap 2.5mg, 5mg*	**HTN**: ini 2.5mg PO bid, maint 5-10mg/d div bid, max 20mg/d; ext.rel: 5-20mg PO qd

Nicardipine	EHL 8.6h, Q0 1.0, PRC C, Lact ?
Cardene *Cap 20mg, 30mg; Inj 2.5mg/ml* **Cardene SR** *Cap ext.rel 30mg, 45mg, 60mg* **Generics** *Cap 20mg, 30mg*	**HTN crisis**: ini 5mg/h IV incr prn by 2.5mg/h q5-15min, max 15mg/h; **HTN**: ini 20mg PO tid, maint 20-40mg tid; ext.rel.: ini 30mg PO bid, maint 30-60mg PO bid, max 120mg/d; **chronic stable AP**: ini 20mg PO tid, maint 20-40mg tid; DARF: not req

Nifedipine	EHL no data, Q0 1.0, PRC C, Lact +
Adalat CC *Tab ext.rel 30mg, 60mg, 90mg* **Afeditab CR** *Tab ext.rel 30mg, 60mg* **Procardia** *Cap 10mg, 20mg* **Procardia XL** *Tab ext.rel 30mg, 60mg, 90mg* **Generics** *Tab ext.rel 30mg, 60mg,* *Cap 10mg, 20mg*	**HTN**: ext.rel: ini 30-60mg PO qd, max 120mg/d; **angina pectoris**: ini 10mg PO tid, maint 10-20mg tid; ext.rel: ini 30-60mg PO qd, max 120mg/d; DARF: not req

Nisoldipine	EHL 7-12h, Q0 1.0, PRC C, Lact ?
Sular *Tab ext.rel 8.5mg, 17mg, 25.5mg, 34mg* **Generics** *20mg, 30mg, 40mg*	**HTN**: ini17- 20mg PO qd, maint 34-40mg qd, max 60mg/d; DARF: not req

5.6.2   CCBs: Non–dihydropyridines

MA: blockage of inflow of calcium ions;
EF: neg. inotropic and chronotropic effect, myocardial O_2 consumption ↓, vasodilation (afterload ↓, preload unchanged), AV conduction time ↑, AV refractory period↑;
AE: AV block, bradycardia, cardiac arrest, hypotension, ankle edema;
CI: AV block II°–III°, SA block, bradycardia, hypersensitivity to drug

Diltiazem	EHL 3-6.6h, Q0 >0.9, PRC C, Lact -
Cardizem *Tab* 30mg, 60mg, 90mg, 120mg, *Inj* 25mg/vial, 100mg/vial, 5mg/ml **Cardizem CD** *Cap ext.rel* 180mg, 240mg, 300mg **Cardizem SR** *Cap ext.rel* 60mg, 90mg, 120mg **Cartia XT** *Cap ext.rel* 120mg, 180mg, 240mg, 300mg **Taztia XT** *Tab ext.rel* 120mg, 180mg, 240mg, 300mg, 360mg **Tiazac** *Cap ext.rel* 120mg, 180mg, 240mg, 300mg, 360mg, 420mg **Generics** *Tab* 30mg, 60mg, 90mg, 120mg, *Tab ext.rel* 120mg, 180mg, 240mg, *Cap ext.rel* 60mg, 90mg, 120mg, 180mg, 240mg, 300mg, *Inj* 5mg/ml	**Chronic stable and vasospastic AP:** ini 30mg PO qid, max 360mg/d; ext.rel: 120-480mg qd, max 540mg/d; **HTN:** ini 60-120mg PO bid, maint 120-180mg bid, max 360mg/d; ext.rel: 240-360mg PO qd; **AF:** ini 0.25mg/kg IV over 2min, rep prn after 15min with 0.35mg/kg; continuous inf: 5-15mg/h; DARF: not req

Verapamil	EHL 4-12h, Q0 >0.8, PRC C, Lact +
Calan *Tab* 40mg, 80mg, 120mg **Covera-HS** *Tab ext.rel* 180mg, 240mg **Isoptin** *Tab* 40mg, 80mg, 120mg, *Inj* 2.5mg/ml **Isoptin SR** *Tab ext.rel* 120mg, 180mg, 240mg **Verelan** *Cap ext.rel* 120mg, 180mg, 240mg, 360mg **Verelan PM** *Cap ext.rel* 100mg, 200mg, 300mg **Generics** *Tab ext.rel* 120mg, 180mg, 240mg, *Tab* 40mg, 80mg, 120mg, *Cap ext.rel* 120mg, 180mg, 240mg, *Inj* 2.5mg/ml	**HTN:** ext.rel: 120-240mg PO qd-bid **chronic stable AP:** ext.rel: 180-360mg PO qd, max 480mg/d; **SVT:** 5-10mg IV over 2min, rep after 15-30min prn; continuous inf: 5mg/h IV; **AF:** 240-480mg PO div tid-qid; **CH** 1-15 y: **arrhythmias:** 0.1-0.3mg/kg IV; DARF: not req

5.7 Adrenergic Inhibitors

5.7.1 Central Acting Alpha Agonists

MA (clonidine, guanabenz, methyldopa): stimulation of central α_2-receptors (presynaptic effect) ⇒ release of noradrenaline ↓, postsynaptic effect ⇒ peripheral sympathetic tone ↓, release of renin ↓, (⇒ inhibition of renin-angiotensin-aldosterone-system); additional agonistic effect on imidazole-receptor;
EF (clonidine, guanabenz, methyldopa): BP ↓ due to reduction of peripheral resistance, stroke volume and cardiac output;
AE (clonidine, guanabenz): AV block, bradycardia, drowsiness, oral dryness;
CI (clonidine, guanabenz): bradycardia

Clonidine	EHL 12-16h, Q0 0.4, PRC C, Lact ?
Catapres Tab 0.1mg, 0.2mg, 0.3mg, Film (ext.rel, TD) 0.1mg/24h, 0.2mg/24h, 0.3mg/24h **Duraclon** Inj 0.1mg/ml, 0.5mg/ml **Generics** Tab 0.1mg, 0.2mg, 0.3mg	**HTN:** ini 0.1 mg PO bid, maint 0.2-0.6mg/d div bid, max 2.4mg/d; TTS: ini 0.1mg/24h patch, max 0.6mg/24h **CH HTN:** ini 5-10μg/kg/d PO div bid-tid, max 0.9mg/d; DARF: not req

Guanabenz	EHL 6h, PRC C, Lact ?
Generics Tab 4mg, 8mg	**HTN:** ini 4mg PO bid, incr by 4-8mg/d at 1-2 wk intervals, max 96mg/d

Methyldopa	EHL 1.7h, Q0 0.4, PRC B, Lact +
Generics Tab 125mg, 250mg, 500mg, Inj 50mg/ml	**HTN:** ini 250mg PO bid-tid, maint 500-2000mg/d div bid-qid; 250-500mg IV q6h; **CH HTN:** 10mg/kg/d PO div bid-qid, max 65 mg/kg/d; 20-40mg/kg/d IV div qid; DARF: GFR (ml/min) >50: q8h; 10-50: q8-12h; <10: q12-24h

5.7.2 Alpha Adrenergic Blockers

MA: reversible blockage of α_1-receptor;
MA (phenoxybenzamine): irreversible blockage of α_1/α_2-receptor;
EF: vasodilation, pre- and afterload ↓
AE: reflex tachycardia (not prazosin), arrhythmia, postural HT, fatigue, nausea, dyspepsia, diarrhea;
"adverse epinephrine effect": epinephrine → vasodilation and BP ↓ when α receptors are blocked due to β-mimetic effect;
AE (Prazosin): "first-dose phenomenon": postural HT after first dose ⇒ slow increase in dosage;
CI: hypersensitivity to drug;
CI (doxazosin, prazosin) hypersensitivity to quinazolines;
CI (phentolamine): myocardial infarction or history of, coronary insufficiency, angina, HT, hypersensitivity to sulfites

Doxazosin	EHL 8.8-22h, Q0 0.95, PRC C, Lact ?
Cardura Tab 1mg, 2mg, 4mg, 8mg **Generics** Tab 1mg, 2mg, 4mg, 8mg	**HTN** (not first line): ini 1mg PO qd, max 16mg/d

Phenoxybenzamine	EHL 24h, PRC C, Lact ?
Dibenzyline Cap 10mg	**Pheochromocytoma:** ini 10mg PO bid, incr slowly qod prn up to 20-40mg bid-tid, max 120mg/d

Phentolamine	EHL 19min, PRC C, Lact ?
Regitine Inj 5mg/vial Generics Inj 5mg/vial	**Pheochromocytoma surgery:** 5mg IV/IM 1-2h prior to surgery, 5mg IV during surgery prn; **CH pheochromocytoma surgery:** 1mg IV/IM 1-2h prior to surgery, 1mg IV during surgery prn

Prazosin	EHL 2-4h, Q0 1.0, PRC C, Lact ?
Minipress Cap 1mg, 2mg, 5mg Generics Cap 1mg, 2mg, 5mg	**HTN:** ini 1mg PO qd, maint 6-15mg/d div bid, max 20mg/d; **CH HTN:** ini 5µg/kg PO as 1x dose; maint 25-150µg/kg/d div q6h, max 0.4 mg/kg/d, DARF: not req

Terazosin	EHL 9-12h, Q0 0.95, PRC C, Lact ?
Hytrin Cap 1mg, 2mg, 5mg, 10mg, Tab 1mg, 2mg, 5mg, 10mg Generics Cap 1mg, 2mg, 5mg, 10mg	**HTN:** ini 1mg PO hs, maint 1-5mg PO qd or div bid, max 20mg/d; DARF: not req

5.7.3 Peripheral Acting Adrenergic Blockers

MA: inhibition of vesicular storage of catecholamines; **EF:** peripheral resistance ↓ (afterload) ⇒ BP ↓, HR ↓, cardiac output ↓; **AE:** depression, gut motility↑, bradycardia, postural HT, stuffy nose **CI:** Hypersensitivity to drug, depression or history of, active peptic ulcer disease, ulcerative colitis, patients receiving electroconvulsive therapy

Reserpine	EHL 50-100h, PRC C, Lact -
Serpalan Tab 0.1mg, 0.25mg Generics Tab 0.1mg, 0.25mg	**HTN:** ini 0.5mg/d PO for 1-2wk, then reduce to 0.1-0.25mg/d PO qd; DARF: GFR (ml/min) >10: 100%; <10: not rated

5.8 Direct Vasodilators

MA/EF: direct effect on the smooth muscles of the small arteries and arterioles ⇒ peripheral resistance ↓ (afterload) ⇒ BP ↓; **MA** (fenoldopam): selective postsynaptic dopamine-1 (DA-1) receptor agonist; **MA** (nesiritide): recombinant human B-type natriuretic peptide ⇒ arterial and venous vasodilation ⇒ PCWP ↓, BP ↓; **AE** (direct vasodilators): HT, Na+, H_2O retention, tachycardia, dizziness, headache; **AE** (hydralazine): GI disturbance, blood dyscrasias; **AE** (nitroprusside): cyanide poisoning; **AE** (iloprost): vasodilation, flushing, increased cough, headache, trismus, N/V, HT, flu syndrome, heart failure, chest pain, renal failure, tachycardia, dyspnea, edema; **AE** (minoxidil): hypertrichosis, pericardial effusion, changes in T wave; **AE** (nesiritide): HT, ventricular tachycardia, angina pectoris, bradycardia, headache, abdominal pain, insomnia, dizziness, anxiety, nausea, vomiting; **CI** (eoprostenol) congestive heart failure due to LV systolic dysfunction, hypersensitivity to drug; **CI** (iloprost): no known CI; **CI** (nesiritide): cardiogenic shock, BP < 90mm Hg; **CI** (nitroprusside): compensated HTN (aortic coarctation, AV shunt), high output failure, metabolic acidosis, congenital optic atrophy, tobacco amblyopia **CI** (minoxidil): pheochromocytoma, pulmonary HTN with mitral stenosis, hypersensitivity to drug

Epoprostenol	EHL 3-5min, PRC B, Lact ?
Flolan *Inj 0.5mg/vial, 1.5mg/vial* **Generics** *Inj 0.5mg/vial, 1.5mg/vial*	**Primary pulmonary HTN:** 2ng/kg/min IV, incr by 2ng/kg/min q15min
Fenoldopam	EHL 5-10min, PRC B, Lact ?
Corlopam *Inj 10mg/ml* **Generics** *Inj 10mg/ml*	**Malignant HTN:** ini 0.1 µg/kg/min IV, incr q 15-20min by increments of 0.05-0.1µg/kg/min prn to 1.6µg/kg/min
Hydralazine	EHL 3-5h, PRC C, Lact +
Generics *Tab 10mg, 25mg, 50mg, 100mg, Inj 20mg/ml*	**HTN emergencies:** 10-20mg IV, 20-40mg IM, rep prn; **HTN:** ini 10mg PO qid for 2-4d, incr to 25mg qid, then 50mg qid, max 400mg/d; **CH HTN emergency:** 0.1-0.5mg/kg IM/IV; **CH HTN:** 0.75-1mg/kg/d PO div q4-6h
Iloprost	EHL 20-30min, PRC C, Lact ?
Ventavis *Sol (inhal) 10µg/1ml; 20µg/2ml*	**Pulmonary HTN:** first dose 2.5µg inhaled, if well tolerated 5µg/dose, 6-9 doses/d, max 45µg/d
Minoxidil	EHL 2.3-28.9h, PRC C, Lact +
Generics *Tab 2.5mg, 10mg*	**Severe HTN:** ini 5mg PO qd, incr to 10-40 mg/d div bid; **CH <12 y:** ini 0.2mg/kg PO qd, incr q3d up to 0.25-1mg/kg/d qd or div bid, max 50mg/d
Nesiritide	EHL 18min, PRC C , Lact ?
Natrecor *Inj 1.5mg/vial*	**Acutely decompensated heart failure:** ini 2µg/kg IV over 1min, then 0.01µg/kg/min
Nitroprusside sodium	EHL 3-4min, Q0 1.0 (0.01)
Nitropress *Inj 25mg/ml, 50mg/vial* **Generics** *Inj 25mg/ml*	**HTN emergencies:** ini 0.3µg/kg/min IV, incr slowly to 10µg/kg/min; DARF: not req
Treprostinil	EHL 2-4h, PRC B, Lact ?
Remodulin *Inj 1mg/ml, 2.5mg/ml, per 5mg/ml, 10mg/ml*	**Pulmonary arterial HTN:** ini 1.25ng/kg/min SC, incr. by 1.25ng/kg/min per wk for the first 4wk, then incr. by max. 2.5ng/kg/min; max 40ng/kg/min

5.9   Pulmonary Arterial Antihypertensives

MA/EF (ambrisentan): specific/competitive antagonist at endothelin receptor types ETL ⇒ inhibition of endothelin-1 effects ⇒ pulmonary artery pressure↓;

MA/EF (bosentan): specific/competitive antagonist at endothelin receptor types ETA and ETB ⇒ inhibition of endothelin-1 effects ⇒ pulmonary artery pressure↓;

MA/EF (sildenafil, tadalafil): inhibition of phospho-diesterase type 5 (PDE5) ⇒ cGMP↑ ⇒ relaxation of pulmonary vascular smooth muscle cells ⇒ pulmonary artery pressure↓

AE (ambrisentan): headache, palpitations, peripheral edema, abdominal pain, constipation, liver injury, anemia, nasopharyngitis, sinusitis, dyspnea, nasal congestion, flushing, birth defects;

AE (bosentan): headache, nasopharyngitis, HT, flushing, edema, liver injury;

AE (sildenafil): headache, insomnia, paresthesias, MI, sudden cardiac death, arrhythmias, flushing, epistaxis, rhinitis, sinusitis, retinal hemorrhage, dyspepsia, diarrhea, gastritis, myalgia, worsening dyspnea, erythema, pyrexia

AE (tadalafil): headache, myalgia, nasopharyngitis, flushing, respiratory infection, extremity pain, nausea, back pain, dyspepsia, rhinitis/sinusitis

CI (ambrisentan): hypersensitivity to ambrisentan; pregnancy, moderate-severe hepatic impairment

CI (bosentan): pregnancy, coadministration with cyclosporine A, glyburide; moderate to severe liver impairment

CI (sildenafil): hypersensitivity to sildenafil; pulmonary veno-occlusive disease; coadministration with nitrates, ritonavir

CI (tadalafil): hypersensitivity to tadalafil, coadministration with nitrates

Ambrisentan	EHL 9h, PRC X, Lact ?
Letairis Tab 5mg, 10mg	Pulmonary arterial HTN (WHO II-III): ini 5mg PO qd may incr. to 10mg qd
Bosentan	EHL 5h, PRC X, Lact -
Tracleer Tab 62.5mg, 125mg	Pulmonary arterial HTN (WHO III-IV): ini 62.5mg PO bid f. 4wk, then 125mg bid;DARF: not req
Sildenafil	EHL 4h, PRC B, Lact ?
Revatio Tab 20mg; Inj 10mg/12.5ml	Pulmonary arterial HTN (WHO I): 20mg PO tid, max 60mg/d; 10mg IV q8h; DARF: not req
Tadalafil	EHL 15-35h, PRC B, Lact ?
Adcirca Tab 20mg	Pulmonary arterial HTN (WHO I): 40mg PO qd; DARF: GFR (ml/min) 31-80: ini 20mg, may incr to 40mgd; <30: avoid use

5.10 Diuretics

5.10.1 Thiazide Diuretics

MA: inhibition of reabsorption of Na^+, Cl^-/H_2O in the distal convoluted tubule, secretion of $K^+\uparrow$;
EF: elimination of Na^+, Cl^-, $H_2O/K^+\downarrow$, excretion of $Ca^{2+}/PO_4^{3-}\downarrow$
AE: $K^+\downarrow$, $Ca^{++}\downarrow$, hyperuricemia, thrombosis, anemia, Gluc $\uparrow$;
CI: anuria, renal insufficiency, sulphonamides hypersensitivity, hepatic coma

Chlorothiazide	EHL 45–120min, PRC C, Lact +
Diuril *Sol (oral) 50mg/ml, Inj 500mg/vial* **Generics** *Tab 250mg, 500mg*	**Edema, HTN:** 0.5–1g/d PO/IV qd or div bid; **CH** 6mo–2y: 10–20mg/kg/d PO qd or div bid, max 375mg/d; **CH** 2–12 y: 1g/d PO qd; **DARF:** GFR (ml/min) 10–50: ineffective, <10: not rec

Chlorthalidone	EHL 40–89h, PRC B, Lact ?
Thalitone *Tab 15mg* **Generics** *Tab 25mg, 50mg*	**HTN:** 12.5–25mg PO qd, maint 12.5–50mg/d; **edema:** ini 30–60mg PO qd or 60mg qod, incr prn to 90–120mg/d

Hydrochlorothiazide	EHL 10–12h, Q0 0.05, PRC B, Lact +
Microzide *Cap 12.5mg* **Oretic** *Tab 50mg* **Generics** *Tab 12.5mg, 25mg, 50mg, Sol (oral) 50mg/5ml*	**Edema:** 25–100mg PO qd or qod; **HTN:** ini 12.5–25mg PO qd, maint 12.5–50mg/d; **CH** 1–2mg/kg/d PO qd or div bid

Indapamide	EHL 14–15h, Q0 0.95, PRC B, Lact ?
Generics *Tab 1.25mg, 2.5mg*	**HTN:** ini 1.25mg PO qd, incr prn, max 5mg/d; **edema:** 2.5–5mg PO qd

Metolazone	EHL 8–14h, PRC B, Lact +
Zaroxolyn *Tab 2.5mg, 5mg, 10mg* **Generics** *Tab 2.5mg, 5mg, 10mg*	**Edema:** 5–10mg PO qd, max 20mg/d; **HTN:** ini 2.5–5mg PO qd, maint 5–20mg/d (Zar.); 0.5–1mg PO qd (Mykrox)

5.10.2 Loop Diuretics

MA/EF: inhibition of the reabsorption of Na^+, Cl^-, K^+/H_2O, primarily in the ascending limb of the loop of Henle ⇒ increased elimination of Na^+, Cl^-, K^+, H_2O, Ca^{2+} and Mg^{2+};
AE: K^+↓, Ca^{++}↓, HT, hyperuricemia, thrombosis, reversible hearing loss;
CI: severe electrolyte depletion, hypovolemia, oliguria/anuria, hepatic coma, hypersensitivity to the drug

Bumetanide	EHL 1-1.5h, Q0 0.35, PRC C, Lact ?
Generics Tab 0.5mg, 1mg, 2mg, Inj 0.25mg/ml	**Edema:** 0.5-2mg PO qd, rep prn doses at 4-5h intervals, max 10mg/d; 0.5-1mg IV/IM, rep prn at 2-3h intervals, max 10mg/d DARF: not req

Ethacrynic acid	EHL 1-4h, Q0 0.75, PRC B, Lact -
Edecrin Tab 25mg, Inj 50mg/vial	**Edema:** 50-200mg/d PO; 0.5-1mg/kg IV, max 100mg/d; **CH** ini 25mg PO, incr prn q2-3d by 25mg, max 2-3mg/kg/d

Furosemide	EHL 30-120min, Q0 0.3, PRC C, Lact ?
Lasix Tab 20mg, 40mg, 80mg **Generics** Tab 20mg, 40mg, 80mg, Sol (oral) 10mg/ml, 40mg/5ml, Inj 10mg/ml	**Edema:** ini 20-80mg PO or 20-40mg IV, incr by 20-40mg q6-8h prn, max 600mg/d; **HTN:** ini 20-40mg PO bid, incr prn; **CH** ini 2mg/kg IV/IM/PO, incr by 1-2mg q6-8h until desired effect is achieved, max 6mg/kg/dose

Torsemide	EHL 3-6h, PRC B, Lact ?
Demadex Tab 5mg, 10mg, 20mg, 100mg, Inj 10mg/ml **Generics** Tab 5mg, 10mg, 20mg, 100mg	**Edema:** ini 10-20mg IV/PO qd, incr prn by doubling the dose, max 200mg qd; **HTN:** 5-10mg PO qd

5.10.3 Potassium-sparing Diuretics

MA (amiloride, triamterene): inhibition of the reabsorption of Na^+, Cl^- and H_2O as well as inhibition of the K^+-secretion in the distal convoluted tubule;
EF: elimination of Na^+, Cl^- and H_2O ↑, K^+ elimination ↓;
AE (amiloride, triamterene): hyperkalemia, metabolic acidosis, megaloblastic anemia;
CI (amiloride): hyperkalemia, renal insufficiency, anuria, use of other antikaliuretics/K salts;
CI (triamterene): hyperkalemia, renal insufficiency

Amiloride	EHL 6-9h, Q0 0.25, PRC B, Lact ?
Midamor Tab 5mg **Generics** Tab 5mg	**Edema/HTN:** ini 5mg PO qd in combination with another diuretic, max 20mg/d

Triamterene	EHL 1.5-2.5h, Q0 0.8, PRC D, Lact -
Dyrenium Cap 50mg, 100mg	**Edema with cirrhosis, nephrotic syndrome, heart failure:** 50-100mg PO bid, max 300mg/d

5.10.4 Aldosterone Antagonists

MA: blocks the binding of aldosterone to the mineralocorticoid receptor;
AE (eplerenone): hyperkalemia, headache, dizziness, diarrhea, abdominal pain;
AE (spironolactone): hyperkalemia, gynecomastia, impotence, amenorrhea, hirsutism, voice disorders, skin disorders, N/V/D, gastric bleeding, agranulocytosis, fever, urticaria, cutaneous eruptions, anaphylactic reactions, vasculitis, fever, mental confusion, headache, renal dysfunction;
CI (eplerenone): hyperkalemia > 5.5mEq/l, type 2 diabetes with microalbuminuria, GFR <50ml/min, combination with strong CYP3A-inhibitors (ketoconazole, itraconazole), potassium-sparing diuretics;
CI (spironolactone): anuria, acute renal insufficiency, K$^+$ ↑

Eplerenone	EHL 4-6 h, PRC B, Lact ?
Inspra *Tab 25mg, 50mg* **Generics** *Tab 25, 50mg*	HTN: ini 50mg PO qd, incr prn after 4wk to 50mg bid; DARF: GFR (ml/min) <50: CI

Spironolactone	EHL 1.3-1.4h, Q0 1.0, PRC D, Lact +
Aldactone *Tab 25mg, 50mg, 100mg* **Generics** *Tab 25mg, 50mg, 100mg*	**Edema with heart failure, cirrhosis, nephrotic syndrome:** ini 100mg PO qd or div bid, incr prn until diuretic effect is achieved, max 200mg/d; **HTN:** 50-100mg PO qd or div bid; **CH** 1-3mg/kg/d PO

5.10.5 Potassium-sparing Diuretics: Combinations

HCTZ + Amiloride	PRC B, Lact -
Generics *Tab 50 + 5mg*	HTN, edema: 50+5 - 100+10mg PO qd

HCTZ + Spironolactone	PRC C, Lact ?
Aldactazide *Tab 25 + 25mg, 50 + 50mg* **Generics** *Tab 25 + 25mg*	**Edema:** 25+25 - 200+200mg PO qd or div bid **HTN:** 50+50 - 100+100mg PO qd or div bid

HCTZ + Triamterene	PRC D, Lact -
Dyazide *Cap 25 + 37.5mg* **Maxzide** *Tab 25 + 37.5mg, 50 + 75mg* **Generics** *Cap 25 + 37.5mg, 25 + 50mg, 50 + 75mg*	**HTN, edema:** 25+37.5 - 50+75mg PO qd or div bid

5.10.6 Diuretics: Carbonic Anhydrase Inhibitors

MA/EF: noncompetitive inhibition of the enzyme carbonic anhydrase ⇒ urine volume ↑, urinary excretion of bicarbonate/sodium ↑ ⇒ metabolic acidosis;
AE: taste disturbance, paresthesia, metabolic acidosis, tinnitus;
CI: hypersensitivity to acetazolamide, sulfonamides or thiazides, Na$^+$↓, K$^+$↓, severe liver or renal impairment, hyperchloremic acidosis, suprarenal gland failure

Acetazolamide	EHL 4-8h, PRC C, Lact ?
Diamox *Cap ext.rel 500mg, Inj 500mg/vial* **Generics** *Tab 125mg, 250mg, Inj 500mg/vial*	**Acute glaucoma:** 250mg IV q4h; 250mg PO qd-qid; **heart failure:** 250-375mg PO qod; **mountain sickness:** 0.5-1g PO div bid-tid, ini 24-48h before ascent, continue for 48h at high altitudes

5.11 Antihypertensive Combinations

Amlodipine + Benazepril	PRC D, Lact ?
Lotrel *Cap* 2.5 + 10mg, 5 + 10mg, 5 + 20mg, 5 + 40mg, 10 + 20mg, 10 + 40mg **Generics** *Cap* 2.5 + 10mg, 5 + 10mg, 5 + 20mg, 5 + 40mg, 10 + 20mg	HTN: 2.5+10 - 10+40mg PO qd; DARF: GFR (ml/min) >30: 100%, <30: not rec

Amlodipine + Olmesartan	PRC C(1st trim.), D(2nd, 3rd trim.), Lact ?
Azor *Tab* 5 + 20mg, 5 + 40mg, 10 + 20mg, 10 + 40mg	HTN: 5+20 - 10+40mg PO qd; DARF: not req

Amlodipine + Olmesartan + HCTZ	PRC D, Lact ?
Tribenzor *Tab* 5 + 20 + 12.5mg, 5 + 40 + 12.5mg, 5 + 40 + 25mg, 10 + 40 + 12.5mg, 10 + 40 + 25mg	HTN: 1 Tab PO qd; use same doses of each component if replacement tx, max 10+40+25mg; DARF: GFR (ml/min) <30: not recommended

Amlodipine + Telmisartan	PRC C(1st trim.), D(2nd, 3rd trim.), Lact ?
Twynsta *Tab* 5 + 40mg, 5 + 80mg, 10 + 40mg, 10 + 80mg	HTN: 5+40 - 10+80mg PO qd; DARF: severe RF: titrate slowly

Amlodipine + Valsartan	PRC C(1st trim.), D(2nd, 3rd trim.), Lact ?
Exforge *Tab* 5 + 160mg, 5 + 320mg, 10 + 160mg, 10 + 320mg	HTN: 5+160 - 10+320mg PO qd; DARF: caution advised in severe RF

Amlodipine + Valsartan + HCTZ	PRC D Lact
Exforge HCT *Tab* 5 + 160 +12.5mg, 5 + 160 + 25mg, 10 + 160 + 12.5mg, 10 + 160 + 25mg, 10 + 320 + 25mg	HTN: 5+160+12.5 - 10+320+25mg PO qd; DARF GFR (ml/min) >30: avoid use

Atenolol + Chlorthalidone	PRC D, Lact
Tenoretic *Tab* 50 + 25mg, 100 + 25mg **Generics** *Tab* 50 + 25mg, 100 + 25mg	HTN: 50+25 - 100+25mg PO qd; DARF: GFR (ml/min) 15-35: 50mg qd, <15: 50mg qod

Bisoprolol + HCTZ	PRC C, Lact
Ziac *Tab* 2.5 + 6.25mg, 5 + 6.25mg, 10 + 6.25mg **Generics** *Tab* 2.5 + 6.25mg, 5 + 6.25mg, 10 + 6.25mg	HTN: 2.5+6.25 - 20+12.5mg PO qd

Clonidine + Chlorthalidone	PRC C, Lact
Clorpres *Tab* 0.1 + 15mg, 0.2 + 15mg, 0.3 + 15mg	HTN: 0.1+15 - 0.6+30mg PO qd or div bid

Hydralazine + HCTZ	PRC C, Lact
Hydra-Zide *Cap* 25 + 25mg, 50 + 50mg, 100 + 50mg	HTN: 25+25 - 100+50mg PO qd

Metoprolol + HCTZ	PRC C, Lact +
Lopressor HCT Tab 50 + 25mg, 100 + 25mg, 100 + 50mg **Generics** Tab 50 + 25mg, 100 + 25mg, 100 + 50mg	**HTN:** 50+25 - 100+50mg PO qd

Nadolol + Bendroflumethiazide	PRC C, Lact -
Corzide Tab 40 + 5mg, 80 + 5mg **Generics** Tab 40 + 5mg, 80 + 5mg	**HTN:** 40+5 - 80+5mg PO qd; DARF: GFR (ml/min) >50: q24h, 31-50: q24-36h, 10-30: q28-48h, <10: q40-60h

Propranolol + HCTZ	PRC C, Lact ?
Generics Tab 40 + 25mg, Tab 80 + 25mg	**HTN:** 40+25 - 160+50mg PO qd or div bid; ext.rel: 80+50 -160+50mg PO qd

Timolol + HCTZ	PRC C, Lact -
Timolide 10-25 Tab 10 + 25mg	**HTN:** 20+50mg PO qd or div bid

Trandolapril + Verapamil	PRC D, Lact -
Tarka Tab ext.rel 1 + 240mg, 2 + 180mg, 2 + 240mg, 4 + 240mg	**HTN:** 1+180 - 4+480mg PO qd or div bid

5.12   Nitrates

5.12.1   Nitrates: Single Ingredient Drugs

MA: NO relaxes smooth musculature of blood vessels;
EF: preload ↓ through venous pooling, coronary spasmolysis; afterload ↓;
AE: BP ↓, tachycardia, headache, tachyphylaxis (not molsidomine)
CI: hypotension, shock, HOCM, severe anemia, early MI, constrictive pericarditis, pericardial tamponade, head trauma/cerebral hemorrhage, hypovolemia

Isosorbide dinitrate	EHL 4h, Q0 1.0, PRC C, Lact ?
Dilatrate-SR Cap ext.rel 40mg **Isordil** Cap ext.rel 40mg, Tab 10mg, 20mg, 30mg, 40mg, 50mg, Tab (SL) 2.5mg, 5mg, 10mg **Generics** Tab 5mg, 10mg, 20mg, 30mg, Tab (SL) 2.5mg, 5mg, Tab ext.rel 40mg	**Angina pectoris Tx:** 2.5-10mg PO/SL, rep prn q5-10min up to 3 doses in 30min; **angina PRO:** ini 5-20mg PO bid-tid, maint 10-40mg bid-tid; ext.rel: ini 40mg PO bid, max 80mg PO bid; a daily dose-free interv. of 10-14h is advisable to avoid nitrate tolerance; DARF: not req

Isosorbide mononitrate	EHL 6.2 and 6.6h, Q0 0.8, PRC C, Lact ?
Imdur Tab ext.rel 30mg, 60mg, 120mg **ISMO** Tab 20mg **Monoket** Tab 10mg, 20mg **Generics** Tab 10mg, 20mg, Tab ext.rel 30mg, 60mg, 120mg	**Angina pectoris:** 20mg PO bid (8 am and 3 pm); ext.rel: ini 30mg PO qd, incr prn to 120mg/d, max 240mg/d

Nitroglycerin IV	EHL 19-33min, PRC C, Lact ?
Nitro-Bid Inj 5mg/ml **Generics** Inj 0.1mg/ml, 5mg/ml, 10mg/100ml, 20mg/100ml, 40mg/100ml	**Acute Angina pectoris, heart failure:** 5-200µg/min IV; **hypertensive emergency:** ini 10-20µg/min IV, incr to max 100µg/min

Nitroglycerin spray	EHL 2-33min, PRC C, Lact ?
Nitrolingual *Aerosol SL 0.4mg/Spray* **Nitrolingual Pumpspray** *Spray metered SL 0.4mg/Spray*	**Acute Angina pectoris**: 0.4-0.8mg SL, rep prn, max 1.2mg in 15min

Nitroglycerin sublingual	EHL 2-33min, PRC C, Lact ?
Nitrostat *Tab (SL) 0.3mg, 0.4mg, 0.6mg*	**Acute Angina pectoris**: 0.3-0.6mg SL or in the buccal pouch, rep prn q5min up to 3 doses in 15min; **angina PRO**: 0.3-0.6mg 5-10min before activities which might precipitate an acute attack; DARF: not req

Nitroglycerin extended release	EHL 2-33min, PRC C, Lact ?
Nitroglyn *Cap ext.rel 2.5mg, 6.5mg, 9mg, 13mg*	**Angina pectoris PRO**: ini 2.5mg PO bid-tid, incr prn; mind a daily dose-free interval of 10-14h to avoid nitrate tolerance; DARF: not req

Nitroglycerin transdermal	EHL 2-33min, PRC C, Lact ?
Minitran *Film (ext.rel, TD) 0.1, 0.2, 0.4, 0.6mg/h* **Nitro-Dur** *Film (ext.rel, TD) 0.1, 0.2, 0.3, 0.4, 0.6mg/h* **Generics** *Film (ext.rel, TD) 0.2, 0.4, 0.6, 0.8mg/h*	**Angina pectoris PRO**: 0.2-0.4mg/h; patch should remain for 12-14h and then be removed

5.12.2 Nitrates: Combinations

AE (bidil): headache, paresthesia, dizziness, asthenia, chest pain, hypotension, ventricular tachycardia, palpitations, sinusitis, amblyopia, N/V, hyperglycemia, hyperlipidemia, bronchitis, angioedema, lupus-like-syndrome, neutropenia, methemoglobinemia
CI (bidil): hypersens. to bidil, severe hypotension

Isosorbide dinitrate + Hydralazine	PRC C, Lact ?
Bidil *Tab 20mg + 37.5mg*	**Heart failure**: 1Tab PO tid, max 2Tab tid; DARF: not req.

5.13 Other Antianginal Drugs

MA (ranolazine): exact MA unknown; inhibits late sodium current, reducing sodium-induced calcium overload in myocytes;
AE (ranolazine): dizziness, headache, constipation, N/V, palpitations, vertigo, abdominal pain, dry mouth, vomiting, peripheral edema, dyspnea;
CI (ranolazine): pre-existing QT prolongation, hepatic impairment (Child-Pugh Classes A-C), combination with QT prolonging drugs or with potent and moderately potent CYP3A inhibitors, including diltiazem

Ranolazine	EHL 6-22h, PRC C, Lact ?
Ranexa *Tab (ext.rel) 500mg, 1000mg*	**Chronic Angina pectoris Tx**: ini 500mg PO bid, incr prn to 1000mg bid; max 1000mg bid; DARF: blood pressure should be monitored

5.14 Antiarrhythmics

Class IA antiarrhythmics (quinidine, disopyramide, procainamide)
MA/EF: inflow of Na^+ blocked $\Rightarrow$ delayed depolarization, conduction velocity $\downarrow$ (neg. dromotropic), threshold potential of the AV node $\uparrow$ (excitability $\downarrow$), neg. inotropic, K^+outflow blocked $\Rightarrow$ action potential length $\uparrow$, refractory time $\uparrow$;
AE: GI impairment, dizziness, confusion, dysopias, BP $\downarrow$, AV block, tachycardia;
AE (disopyramide): urinary retention, constipation, accommodation impaired, dry mouth;
AE (procainamide): appetite loss, diarrhea, allergic reactions/dermatitis, itching, dizziness, systemic lupus, hypotension, QT interval prolongation;
CI: AV block II°-III°;
CI (quinidine): myasthenia gravis, history of drug induced *torsades*, uncompensated heart failure, junctional or intraventricular conduction delay, prolonged QT interval, digitalis overdose;
CI (disopyramide): shock, extensive myocardial disease, glaucoma, urinary retension, renal failure, intraventricular conduction delay;
CI (procainamide): history of *Torsades de Pointes*, SLE, myasthenia gravis

Class IB antiarrhythmics (lidocaine, mexiletine, tocainide)
MA: Na^+ inflow $\downarrow$, K^+ outflow $\uparrow$, slowed phase 4 depolarization;
EF: excitability $\downarrow$, especially in the ventricles, action potential duration and refractory time in Purkinje fibers $\downarrow$, in atria and ventricles $\uparrow$; high-frequency excitations are filtered out (premature contractions), possible AV conduction time $\uparrow$, negative inotropic effect smaller than class Ia, in high concentrations neg. dromotropic, neg. inotropic;
AE (lidocaine): anxiety, drowsiness, dizziness, nervousness, convulsions, pain at injection site, paresthesia, allergic reaction, N/V;
AE (mexiletine): dizziness, heartburn, lightheadedness, N/V, nervousness, tremors;
CI: AV block II°-III°;
CI (lidocaine): Adam-Stokes syndrome, SA or intraventricular conduction delay;
CI (mexiletine): cardiogenic shock

Class IC antiarrhythmics (flecainide, moricizine, propafenone)
MA: conduction and refractory time $\uparrow$ (AV node and ventricle), no vagolysis
AE: hypotension, AV block, nausea, pro-arrhythmias, cholestatic hepatitis
CI (flecainide): AV block II°-III°, shock, bi- or trifascicular block,
CI (propafenone): sinus or AV dysfunction, bradycardia, severe cardiac insufficiency, bronchospastic disease, severe electrolyte imbalance or hepatic failure

Class II antiarrhythmics see Beta Blockers →192

Class III antiarrhythmics (amiodarone, bretylium, ibutilide, dofetilide, sotalol)
MA/EF: blockade of K^+ channels $\Rightarrow$ action potential length $\uparrow$;
AE (amiodarone): corneal microdeposits, pulmonary fibrosis, hepatic damage, photosensitivity, dysopias, erythema nodosum, hypo- and hyperthyroidism;
AE (bretylium): hypotension, syncope, bradycardia, frequency of arrhythmias $\uparrow$, dizziness, vertigo, N/V
AE (sotalol): see Beta Blockers →192;
CI (amiodarone): AV block II°-III°, bradycardia, thyroid diseases, iodine allergy, acute hepatitis, thyroid dysfunction, pulmonary interstitial abnormalities
CI (bretylium): orthostatic hypotension;
CI (sotalol): see Beta Blockers →192

Class IV antiarrhythmics (verapamil) see Calcium Channel Blockers - Non-Dihydropyridines →200

Other Antiarrhythmics (adenosine, atropine, digoxin →214, epinephrine →191)

MA/EF (adenosine): brief blockade of the AV node ⇒ termination of re-entry tachycardias, neg. chronotropic at the sinus node

MA/EF (atropine): compet. antagonism at muscarinic rec. ⇒ tachycardia, antispasmodic, tear production ↓; sputum, sweating ↓, bronchial secretion ↓, mydriasis, blurred vision

MA/EF (dronedarone): exact MA unknown; exhibits antiarrhythmic properties of all four Vaughn-Williams classes

AE (adenosine): flush, dyspnea, bronchospasm, nausea;

AE (atropine): decrease of sweat production, urinary retention, restlessness, hallucinations, oral dryness, acute glaucoma

AE (dronedarone): elevated creatinine, QT prolongation, diarrhea, asthenia, N/V, pruritus/rash, abdominal pain, bradycardia, dyspepsia

CI (adenosine): AV block II°-III°, sick-sinus, bradycardia

CI (atropine): narrow angle glaucoma, micturition disturbance, prostatic hypertrophy, tachyarrhythmias, pyloric stenosis, thyrotoxicosis, GI obstruction, paralytic ileus, severe ulcerative colitis, toxic megacolon, myasthenia gravis

CI (dronedarone): hypersens. to d., CHF NYHA IV, CHF with recent decompensation NYHA II-III, AV block II-III without pacemaker, sick sinus without pacemaker, bradycardia <50/min, QTc >500 msec before or during therapy, PR interval >280 msec, hypokalemia, hypomagnesemia, severe hepatic impairment, pregnancy, breastfeeding

Adenosine	Class IA, EHL <10s, Q0 1.0, PRC C, Lact ?
Adenocard Inj 3mg/ml **Adenoscan** Inj 3mg/ml **Generics** Inj 3mg/ml	**SVT:** 6mg IV as rapid bolus; if tachycardia persists after 1-2min then 12mg IV; **CH SV arrhythmias conversion:** ini 0.05mg/kg IV as rapid bolus, then 0.05-0.1mg/kg IV, max 12mg/dose; DARF: not req
Amiodarone	Class III, EHL 28-107 days, Q0 1.0, PRC D, Lact -
Cordarone Tab 200mg **Nexterone** Inj 50mg/ml **Pacerone** Tab 100mg, 200mg **Generics** Tab 100mg, 200mg, 400mg, Inj 50mg/ml	**Ventricular arrhythmias:** ini 150mg IV over 10min, then 360mg over 6h (1mg/min), then 540mg IV over 18h (0.5mg/min); or 800-1600mg PO qd for 1-3 wk, then 600-800mg qd for 1 mo, then maint 200-400mg qd; **ACLS: VF/PVT:** 300mg IV, may rep with 150mg; **CH** 5mg/kg IV, rep up to 15mg/kg, max 300mg; DARF: not req
Atropine	EHL 4h, Q0 0.45, PRC C, Lact ?
Atropen Inj 0.25mg sulfate/0.3ml, 0.5mg sulfate/0.7ml, 2mg sulfate/0.7ml	**ACLS: asystole:** 1mg IV may rep q3-5min, max 3mg; **CH** 0.02mg/kg IV, minimum dose ≥ 0.1mg, max 0.5mg/dose, may rep once prn; **bradycardia:** 0.5mg IV, may rep q3-5min, max 3mg
Bretylium	Class III, EHL 6-13.5h, PRC C, Lact ?
Generics Inj 50mg/ml, 100mg/100ml, 200mg/100ml, 400mg/100ml	**VF:** ini 5mg/kg IV, then 10mg/kg if arrhythmia persists, max 30mg/kg IV; continuous suppression: 1-2mg/min IV

Digoxin	EHL 1.3-2.2 days, Q0 0.3, PRC C, Lact +
Digoxin pediatric *Inj 0.1mg/ml* **LanoxiCaps** *Cap 0.05mg, 0.1mg, 0.2mg* **Lanoxin** *Tab 0.125, 0.25mg, Inj 0.25mg/ml* **Lanoxin pediatric** *Inj 0.1mg/ml* **Generics** *Tab 0.125, 0.25mg, Inj 0.25mg/ml*	**AF, heart failure:** ini 0.5mg IV, then 0.25mg q6h for 2 doses; maint 0.125-0.375mg PO/IV qd; **CH** 5-10 y: ini 20-35µg/kg PO div q6-8h, maint 25-35% of loading dose; DARF: see Prod Info
Disopyramide	Class IA, EHL 4-10h, Q0 0.4, PRC C, Lact +
Norpace *Cap 100mg, 150mg* **Norpace CR** *Cap ext.rel 100mg, 150mg* **Generics** *Cap 100, 150mg; Cap ext.rel 150mg*	**Ventric. arrhythmias:** 150mg PO qid; ext.rel: 300mg PO bid; DARF: GFR (ml/min) >40: 100mg qid or 200mg bid; 30-40: 100mg tid; 15-30: 100mg bid; <15: 100mg qd
Dofetilide	Class III, EHL 7.5-10h, PRC C, Lact ?
Tikosyn *Cap 0.125mg, 0.25mg, 0.5mg*	**AF** : 0.5mg PO bid; DARF: GFR (ml/min) >60: 100%, 40-60: 0.25mg bid, 20-40: 0.125 mg bid, <20: contraind.
Dronedarone	EHL 13-19h, PRC X, Lact -
Multaq *Tab 400mg*	**Prevention of AF:** 400mg PO bid; DARF: not req.
Epinephrine	EHL no data, PRC C, Lact ?
Adrenaclick *Inj (IM/SC) 0.15, 0.3mg/delivery* **Epipen Jr.** *Inj (IM) 0.15mg/delivery* **Epipen** *Inj (IM) 0.3mg/delivery* **Twinject** *Inj (IM/SC) 0.15, 0.3mg/delivery* **Generics** *Inj (IM) 0.15mg/delivery*	**ACLS: pulseless cardiac arrest:** 1mg (sol 1:10,000) IV, rep q3-5min prn; 2-2.5mg ET; **CH** 0.01mg/kg IV, max 1mg/kg IV (sol 1:10,000); **anaphylaxis:** 0.3-0.5mg/kg IM, rep q10-15min prn; 0.1mg over 5min IV or 1-4µg/min IV
Flecainide	Class IC, EHL 14h, Q0 0.7, PRC C, Lact +
Tambocor *Tab 50mg, 100mg, 150mg* **Generics** *Tab 50mg, 100mg, 150mg*	**SV/ventricular arrhythmias:** 200-400mg/d PO div bid; **CH** >6 mo: 100-200mg/m²/d PO; DARF: GFR (ml/min) <35: 50mg PO bid
Ibutilide	Class III, EHL 2-12h, PRC C, Lact ?
Corvert *Inj 0.1mg/ml* **Generics** *Inj 0.1mg/ml*	**Conversion of AF:** >60kg: 1mg IV over 10min; <60kg: 0.01mg/kg; rep equal dose if no response after 10min; DARF: not req
Isoproterenol	Group II, EHL 3-7h, PRC C, Lact ?
Isuprel *Inj 0.2mg/ml* **Generics** *0.02mg/ml, Inj 0.2mg/ml;*	**Third degree AV block:** ini 0.02-0.06mg IV, then 2-10 µg/min; **CH third degree AV block:** 0.1-1µg/kg/min IV
Lidocaine	Class IB, EHL 1.5-2h, PRC B, Lact +
Generics *Inj 0.5%, 1%, 1.5%, 2%, 4%, 10%, 20%, Inj 200mg/100ml, 400mg/100ml, 800mg/100ml*	**Ventricular arrhythmia:** ini 50-100mg IV, then 1-4mg/min continuous inf; **CH ventricular arrhythmia:** ini 1mg/kg IV, then 20-50µg/kg/min inf; **anesthesia**
Mexiletine	Class IB, EHL 6-17h, Q0 0.8, PRC C, Lact +
Generics *Cap 150mg, 200mg, 250mg*	**Ventricular arrhythmia:** ini 400mg PO, maint 200mg PO q8h

Procainamide	Class IA, EHL 2.5–8h, PRC C, Lact ?
Generics *Tab ext.rel 250mg, 500mg, 750mg, 1g, Cap 250mg, 375mg, 500mg, Inj 100mg/ml, 500mg/ml*	**Ventricular arrhythmias:** ini 100mg slow IV q5min, max 1g or until arrhythmia is supressed, then 2–6mg/min as continuous inf; 50mg/kg/d PO div q3h (immediate-release products), q6h (sustained release products), q12h (Procanbid)

Propafenone	Class IC, EHL 5–8h, Q0 1.0, PRC C, Lact ?
Rythmol *Tab 150mg, 225mg, 300mg* **Rythmol SR** *Tab ext.rel 225mg, 325mg, 425mg* **Generics** *Tab 150mg, 225mg, 300mg*	**Paroxysmal SVT, paroxysmal AF, ventricular arrhythmias:** ini 150mg PO q8h, incr q3-4d to 225mg q8h, max 900mg/d; DARF: not req

Quinidine gluconate	Class IA, EHL no data, PRC C, Lact ?
Generics *Tab ext.rel 324mg; Inj 80mg/ml*	**Maintenance after conversion of AF:** 324–648 mg PO q8–12h; DARF: not req

Quinidine sulfate	Class IA, EHL no data, PRC C, Lact ?
Generics *Tab 100mg, 200mg, 300mg, Tab ext.rel 300mg*	**Maintenance after conversion of AF:** 200–400mg PO q4–6h; 300–600mg PO q8–12h (ext.rel); **CH** 6mg/kg PO q4–6h; DARF: not req

Sotalol	Class III, EHL 7–18h, Q0 0.015, PRC B, Lact ?
Betapace *Tab 80mg, 120mg, 160mg, 240mg* **Betapace AF** *Tab 80mg, 120mg, 160mg* **Sorine** *Tab 80mg, 120mg, 160mg, 240mg* **Generics** *Tab 80mg, 120mg, 160mg, 240mg*	**AF, ventricular arrhythmia:** ini 80mg PO bid, maint 160–320mg/d div bid; DARF: see Prod Info

5.15 Cardiac Glycosides

MA: inhibition of active Na^+-K^+-transport into heart muscle cells $\Rightarrow$ intracellular Na^+ $\uparrow$ $\Rightarrow$ Na^+-Ca^{2+} exchange $\Rightarrow$ intracellular Ca^{2+} $\uparrow$, vagal nerve activity $\uparrow$, sympathetic activity $\downarrow$
EF: pos. inotropic, stroke volume $\uparrow$, higher efficiency of the insufficient heart, tissue perfusion $\uparrow$, coronary perfusion $\uparrow$, neg. chronotropic and dromotropic, refractory time at SA node $\uparrow$, at the myocardial $\downarrow$, $\Rightarrow$ activation of ectopic pacemakers, pos. bathmotropic
AE: AV block, arrhythmias, extrasystoles, allergic reaction, allergic dermatitis, skin rash, N/V, diarrhea, blurred vision, visual halos, confusion
CI: AV block II°–III°, WPW-syndrome, VT, carotid sinus syndrome, hypertrophic obstructive cardiomyopathy, myocardial ischemia, acute MI, pacemakers, hypercalcemia, hypokalemia, thoracic aortic aneurysm, ventricular fibrillation

Digoxin	EHL 1.3–2.2d, Q0 0.3, PRC C, Lact +
Digoxin pediatric *Inj 0.1mg/ml* **LanoxiCaps** *Cap 0.05mg, 0.1mg, 0.2mg* **Lanoxin** *Tab 0.125, 0.25mg, Inj 0.25mg/ml* **Lanoxin pediatric** *Inj 0.1mg/ml* **Generics** *Tab 0.125, 0.25mg, Inj 0.25mg/ml*	**AF, heart failure:** ini 0.5mg IV, then 0.25mg q6h for 2 doses; maint 0.125–0.375mg PO/IV qd; **CH** 5–10 y: ini 20–35μg/kg PO div q6–8h, maint 25–35% of loading dose; DARF: see Prod Info

Digoxin-Immune Fab	EHL 15–20h, PRC C, Lact +
Digibind *Inj 38mg/vial*	**Digoxin/digitoxin–intoxication:** average-dose: 400mg IV; 40mg will bind 0.5-0.6mg digoxin or digitoxin

5.16   Phosphodiesterase Inhibitors

MA: inhibition of phosphodiesterase ⇒ intracellular accumulation of cAMP ⇒ intracellular Ca^{++} ↑ ⇒ myocardial contractility ↑; **EF:** pos. inotropic effect (stroke volume, cardiac output ↑), pos. chronotropic effect, vasodilation (preload ↓, afterload ↓), bronchodilation
AE: cholestasis, nausea, hypotension, tachyarrhythmias, thrombocytopenia, splenomegaly, vasculitis, myositis, lung infiltration; **CI:** hypersensitivity to drug

Inamrinone (Amrinone)	EHL 4.8–8.3h, PRC C, Lact ?
Amrinone Inj 5mg/ml	**Heart failure:** ini 0.75mg/kg IV over 2–3min, maint 5–10mg/kg/min; after 30min additional 0.75mg/kg IV prn

Milrinone	EHL 1–3h, Q0 0.2, PRC C, Lact ?
Primacor Inj 1mg/ml, 20mg/100ml **Generics** Inj 1mg/ml, 20mg/100ml	**Heart failure:** ini 50μg/kg IV over 10min, maint 0.375–0.75μg/kg/min; **DARF:** GFR (ml/min). 41–50: 0.43*, 31–40: 0.38, 21–30: 0.33*, 11–20: 0.28*, 6–10: 0.23*, <5: 0.2* (* = μg/kg/min)

5.17   Antilipidemics

5.17.1   Bile Acid Sequestrants

MA/EF: intestinal binding of bile acids ⇒ interruption of the biliary cycle ⇒ bile acid production from cholesterol ↑ ⇒ serum cholesterol ↓; LDL-receptor activity ↑ ⇒ LDL-resorp. of the liver ↑ ⇒ serum cholesterol ↓; **AE:** constipation, abdominal discomfort/pain, nausea, diarrhea, resorption failure of drugs and fat-soluble vitamins; **AE (colesevelam):** dyspepsia, constipation;
AE (colestipol): constipation, fat soluble vitamin deficiency, N/V, flatulence, abdominal distention;
AE (cholestyramine): constipation, abdominal discomfort/pain, flatulence, N/V, bleeding tendencies due to hypoprothrombinemia; **CI:** bile duct obstruction; **CI (colesevelam):** bowel obstruction, hypersensitivity to colesevelam; **CI (colestipol):** hypersensitivity to colestipol products, complete biliary obstruction, phenylketonurics; **CI (cholestyramine):** complete biliary obstruction, hyperlipidemia types III, IV, or V, hypersensitivity to bile-sequestering resins

Colesevelam	EHL no data, PRC B, Lact ?
Welchol Tab 625mg; Susp. (oral) 1.875g/packet, 3.75g/packet	**Hypercholesterolemia, DM type 2:** 3 TabPO bid or 6Tabqd; 1.875g packet PO bid or 3.75g qd

Colestipol	EHL no data, PRC , Lact +
Colestid Tab 1g, Gran (oral) 5g/pkt, 5g/scoopful **Flavored Colestid** Gran (oral) 5g/pkt, 5g/scoopful **Generics** Gran (oral) 5g/pkt, 5g/scoopful	**Hypercholesterolemia:** Tab: ini 2g PO qd/bid, max 16g/d; Gran: ini 5g PO qd/bid, incr by 5g increments at 1–2 mo intervals, max 30g/d; **DARF:** not req

Cholestyramine	EHL no data, PRC C, Lact ?
Locholest Powder (oral) 4g/9g **Locholest Light** Powder (oral) 4g/5g **Prevalite** Powder (oral) 4g/5g **Questran** Powder (oral) 4g/9g **Questran Light** Powder (oral) 4g/5g **Generics** Powder (oral) 4g/5g, 4g/9g	**Hypercholesterolemia:** ini 4g PO qd/bid, maint 8–16g/d div bid/qid, max 24g/d **DARF:** not req

5.17.2 Cholesterol Absorption Inhibitors

MA/EF (ezetimibe): inhibition of the intestinal absorption of cholesterol and related phytosterols;
AE (ezetimibe): fatigue, pharyngitis, sinusitis, abd. pain, diarrhea, back pain, arthralgia, cough, viral infection; **CI** (ezetimibe): hypersensitivity to e., hepatic dysfunction

Ezetimibe	EHL 22h, PRC C, Lact
Zetia *Tab 10mg*	**Primary hypercholesterolemia, homozyg. fam. hypercholesterolemia, homozyg. sitosterolemia:** 10mg PO qd, may be administered with an HMG-CoA reductase inhibitor; **mixed hyperlipidemia:** 10mg PO qd with fenofibrate; **DARF:** not req

5.17.3 HMG-CoA Reductase Inhibitors ("Statins")

MA/EF: competitive inhib. of HMG CoA reductase ⇒ intracellular cholesterol synthesis ↓, LDL ↓, HDL ↑;
AE: skin reactions, myopathy, vasculitis, headache, abdom. pain, transaminases ↑, dyssomnia;
AE (atorvastatin): headache, liver enzymes ↑, abdom. pain;
AE (fluvastatin): dyspepsia, diarrhea, abdominal pain, nausea, headache;
AE (lovastatin): headache, rhabdomyolysis, diarrhea, hepatotoxicity;
AE (pitavastatin): myalgia, back pain, diarrhea, constipation, pain in extremity, rhabdomyolysis, liver enzyme abnormalities
AE (pravastatin): GI disturbance, liver enzymes ↑, headache, weakness, flu-like symptoms;
AE (simvastatin): headache, GI upset, rhabdomyolysis, transient HT, liver dysfunction;
CI: hepatic diseases, cholestasis, pregnancy, lactation, myopathy, hypersensitivity to product ingredients;
CI (pitavastatin): hypersensitivity to p., active liver disease, unexplained persistent elevations of transaminases, nursing mothers, pregnancy, coadmin. with cyclosporine
CI (rosuvastatin): coadmin. with cyclosporine

Atorvastatin	EHL 14h, Q0 >0.7, PRC X, Lact -
Lipitor *Tab 10mg, 20mg, 40mg, 80mg*	**Hyperchol., mixed dyslipidemia:** ini 10 mg PO qd, maint 10-80mg PO qd, DARF: not req

Fluvastatin	EHL < 3 h, Q0 1.0, PRC X, Lact -
Lescol *Cap 20mg, 40mg* **Lescol XL** *Tab ext.rel 80mg*	**Hypercholesterolemia:** ini 20-40mg PO qd, max 80mg/d

Lovastatin	EHL no data, Q0 1.0, PRC X, Lact -
Altoprev *Tab ext. rel. 20mg, 40mg, 60mg* **Mevacor** *Tab 20mg, 40mg* **Generics** *tab 10mg, 20mg, 40mg*	**Hypercholesterolemia:** ini 20mg PO qd, maint 10-80mg/d PO

Pitavastatin	EHL 12h, PRC X, Lact -
Livalo *Tab 1mg, 2mg, 4mg*	**Primary Hyperlipidemia, mixed dyslipidemia:** 2mg PO qd, incr prn to max 4mg/d; **DARF:** GFR (ml/min) 30-60, HD: ini 1mg qd, max 2mg/d

Pravastatin	EHL 2.6-3.2 h, Q0 0.55, PRC X, Lact -
Pravachol *Tab 10mg, 20mg, 40mg* **Generics** *Tab 10mg, 20mg, 40mg*	**Hypercholesterolemia:** ini 10-20mg PO qd, maint 10-40mg/d; **DARF:** ini 10mg PO qd

Rosuvastatin	EHL 19h, PRC X, Lact -
Crestor *Tab* 5mg, 10mg, 20mg, 40mg	**Hypercholesterolemia, elevated TG-levels** (Ind see also Prescr.Info): ini 10-20mg PO qd, maint 5-40mg/d; DARF: GFR (ml/min) < 30: ini 5mg PO, max 10mg qd

Simvastatin	EHL no data, Q0 1.0, PRC X, Lact -
Zocor *Tab* 5mg, 10mg, 20mg, 40mg, 80mg **Generics** *Tab* 5mg, 10mg, 20mg, 40mg, 80mg	**Hypercholesterolemia**: ini 20-40mg PO qd, maint 5-80mg/d; DARF: ini 5mg PO qd

5.17.4 Statin Combinations

AE (simvastatin + ezetimibe): myopathy, myalgia, diarrhea, abdominal pain, constipation, fatigue, back pain, elevated transaminases, elevated CK, pancreatitis, hypersensitivity-reaction
AE (lovastatin, simvastatin + niacin): flushing, headache, back pain, diarrhea, nausea, pruritus, hepatotoxicity;
AE (simvastatin + ezetimibe): known hypersensitivity, active liver disease, unexplained elevation in transaminases, pregnancy, nursing mothers
CI (lovastatin, simvastatin + niacin): known hypersensitivity, active liver disease, peptic ulcer disease, arterial bleeding, pregnancy, nursing mothers

Atorvastatin + Amlodipine	EHL no data, PRC X, Lact -
Caduet *Tab* 10 + 2.5mg, 10 + 5mg, 10 + 10mg, 20 + 2.5mg, 20 + 5mg, 20 + 10mg, 40 + 2.5mg, 40 + 5mg, 40 + 10mg, 80 + 10mg	**Hypercholesterolemia + HTN** (IND see also Prescr.Info): ini 10-20mg + 5mg PO qd, adjust dose prn according to LDL-C-level, BP; max. 80 + 10mg qd; DARF: not req

Lovastatin + Niacin	EHL no data, PRC X, Lact -
Advicor *Tab ext.rel* 20 + 500mg, 20 + 1000mg	**Hypercholesterolemia**: ini 20 + 500mg PO qd, maint 20-40 + 500-2000mg/d PO

Simvastatin + Ezetimibe	EHL no data, PRC X, Lact -
Vytorin *Tab* 10 + 10mg, 20 + 10mg, 40 + 10mg, 80 + 10 mg	**Hypercholesterolemia, homozyg. familial hyperchol.**: ini 20 + 10mg PO qd, incr. prn to 80 +10mg according to LDL-C-level; DARF: not req in mild-moderate RF

Simvastatin + Niacin	EHL no data, PRC X, Lact-
Simcor *Tab* 20 + 500mg, 20 + 750mg,20 + 1000mg	**Hypercholesterolemia, hypertriglyceridemia**: ini 20 + 500mg PO qd, incr. niacin dose by 500mg steps q4wk to 20 + 1000mg up to 40 + 2000mg depending on tolerability and lipid levels;

5.18   NCEP ATP III Guidelines

5.18.1   LDL-Goals

Risk Category	LDL-Goals	LDL-level at which to consider drug therapy
CHD or CHD risk equivalents	< 100 mg/dL	≥ 130 mg/dL[2]
≥ 2 risk factors[1]		
10-year-risk 10-20%	<130 mg/dL	≥ 130 mg/dL
10-year-risk <10%	<130 mg/dl	≥ 160 mg/dL
<2 risk factors	<160 mg/dL	≥ 190 mg[3]

1: smoking, HTN, HDL< 40 mg/dL, family history of premature CHD
2: drug optional 100-129 mg/dL; 3: drug optional 160-189 mg/dL

Expert panel on detection, evaluation and treatment of high blood cholesterol in adults; JAMA 2001; 285: 2486-249

NCEP: National Cholesterol Education Program; ATP: Adult Treatment Panel
www.nhlbi.nih.gov/guidelines/cholesterol/index.htm

5.18.2   Fibric Acids

MA/EF: lipoprotein lipase activity ↑ ⇒ triglyc. ↓, LDL ↓, HDL ↑;
AE: myalgia, rhabdomyolysis, N/V, transaminases ↑, cholelithiasis, ventricular dysrhythmia, blood count changes;
AE (fenofibrate): rash, LFT ↑;
AE (gemfibrozil): epigastric pain, xerostomia, diarrhea, myopathy, hepatotox.;
CI: primary biliary cirrhosis, great caution in children;
CI (fenofibrate): severe hepatic or renal disease, gallbladder disease, hypersensitivity to fenofibrate;
CI (gemfibrozil): hypersensitivity to gemfibrozil, gallbladder disease/biliary cirrhosis, severe liver/ kidney disease, type I hyperlipoproteinemia

Fenofibrate	EHL 20-22h, Q0 0.2, PRC C, Lact -
Antara Cap 43mg, 130mg Lipofen Cap 50mg, 100mg, 150mg Tricor Tab 48mg, 145mg Triglide Tab 50mg, 160mg Generics Tab 54mg, 67mg, 134mg, 200mg	**Hypertriglyceridemia, hypercholesterolemia**: ini 50-160mg PO qd, 50mg qd if elderly, incr q4-8wk, max 160mg/d; DARF: GFR (ml/min) 20-50: ini 50mg qd; <20: contraind.

Gemfibrozil	EHL 1.5 h, Q0 1.0, PRC C, Lact -
Lopid Tab 600mg Generics Tab 600mg	**Hypertriglyceridemia**: 600mg PO bid

5.18.3 Nicotinic Acid, Others

MA/EF (niacin): blockage of the triacylglycerol lipase ⇒ lipoprotein lipase activity↑ ⇒ triglycerides ↓, cholesterine↓;
MA/EF (omega-3-acids): reduction of hepatic triglyceride synthesis;
AE (niacin): flush, a sensation of warmth in face, neck, ears, GI disturbance, glucose tolerance↓, fasting blood sugar↑, pruritus, hepatotoxity, feeling of restlessness, headache, HT, rash, tingling, itching, dry skin;
AE (omega-3-acids): eruct., infection, flu syndrome, dyspepsia, taste changes, back pain, rash, angina, pain;
CI (niacin): acute CVS failure, hypersensitivity to niacin, active liver/peptic ulcer disease;
CI (omega-3-acids): hypersensitivity to omega-3-acids; use cautiousness in hypersensitivity to fish

Niacin	EHL 10h, PRC C, Lact ?
Niacor *Tab 500mg* **Niaspan** *Tab ext.rel. 500mg, 750mg, 1g* **Generics** *Tab 500mg*	**Hyperlipoproteinemia/hyperlipidemia**: ini 100mg PO tid incr slowly to 3g/d, max 6g/d; ext.rel.: 375mg PO qd for 1wk, then 500mg PO qd for 1wk, then 750mg PO qd for 1wk, then 1000mg PO qd; max 2g/d
Omega-3-acid ethyl esters	EHL no data, PRC C, Lact ?
Lovaza *Cap 1g*	**Hypertriglyceridemia**: 4g/d PO qd or div bid

Links to Guidelines

Heart Disease and Stroke Statistics-2010 Update
http://circ.ahajournals.org/cgi/reprint/CIRCULATIONAHA.109.192667

ACCF/SCCT/ACR/AHA/ASE/ASNC/NASCI/SCAI/SCMR 2010 Appropriate Use Criteria for Cardiac Computed Tomography
http://circ.ahajournals.org/cgi/reprint/CIR.0b013e3181fcae66

Guidelines for the Prevention of Stroke in Patients With Stroke or Transient Ischemic Attack
http://stroke.ahajournals.org/cgi/reprint/STR.0b013e3181f7d043

2010 International Consensus on Cardiopulmonary Resuscitation and Emergency Cardiovascular Care Science With Treatment Recommendations
http://circ.ahajournals.org/content/vol122/16_suppl_2/

2010 American Heart Association Guidelines for Cardiopulmonary Resuscitation and Emergency Cardiovascular Care Science
http://circ.ahajournals.org/content/vol122/18_suppl_3/

Acute Heart Failure Syndromes: Emergency Department Presentation, Treatment and Disposition: Current Approaches and Future Aims
http://circ.ahajournals.org/cgi/reprint/CIR.0b013e3181f9a223

Testing of Low-Risk Patients Presenting to the Emergency Department With Chest Pain
http://circ.ahajournals.org/cgi/reprint/CIR.0b013e3181ec61df

ADA/AHA/ACCF Aspirin for Primary Prevention of Cardiovascular Events in People With Diabetes
http://circ.ahajournals.org/cgi/reprint/CIR.0b013e3181e3b133

ACCF/ACR/AHA/NASCI/SCMR 2010 Expert Consensus Document on Cardiovascular Magnetic Resonance
http://circ.ahajournals.org/cgi/reprint/CIR.0b013e3181d44a8f

ACCF/ACR/AHA/NASCI/SAIP/SCAI/SCCT 2010 Expert Consensus Document on Coronary Computed Tomographic Angiography
http://circ.ahajournals.org/cgi/reprint/CIR.0b013e3181d4b618

ACC/AHA Guideline Based on 2010 Guidelines for the Diagnosis and Management of Patients With Thoracic Aortic Disease
http://circ.ahajournals.org/cgi/reprint/CIR.0b013e3181d47d48

2009 Focused Updates: ACC/AHA Guidelines for the Management of Patients With ST-Elevation Myocardial Infarction (Updating the 2004 Guideline and 2007 Focused Update) and ACC/AHA/SCAI Guidelines on Percutaneous Coronary Intervention (Updating the 2005 Guideline and 2007 Focused Update)
http://circ.ahajournals.org/cgi/reprint/CIRCULATIONAHA.109.192663

2009 ACCF/AHA Focused Update on Perioperative Beta Blockade
http://circ.ahajournals.org/cgi/reprint/CIRCULATIONAHA.109.192689

ACCF/ASNC/ACR/AHA/ASE/SCCT/SCMR/SNM 2009 Appropriate Use Criteria for Cardiac Radionuclide Imaging
http://circ.ahajournals.org/cgi/reprint/CIRCULATIONAHA.109.192519

2009 Focused Update: ACCF/AHA Guidelines for the Diagnosis and Management of Heart Failure in Adults
http://circ.ahajournals.org/cgi/reprint/CIRCULATIONAHA.109.192064

AHA/ACCF/HRS Recommendations for the Standardization and Interpretation of the Electrocardiogram
http://circ.ahajournals.org/cgi/reprint/CIRCULATIONAHA.108.191098

2008 Focused Update Incorporated Into the ACC/AHA 2006 Guidelines for the Management of Patients With Valvular Heart Disease
http://circ.ahajournals.org/cgi/reprint/CIRCULATIONAHA.108.190748

Resistant Hypertension: Diagnosis, Evaluation, and Treatment
http://hyper.ahajournals.org/cgi/reprint/HYPERTENSIONAHA.108.189141

Guidelines for Management of Patients With Atrial Fibrillation
http://content.onlinejacc.org/cgi/content/full/48/4/854

Guidelines for Management of Patients with Chronic Stable Angina
http://content.onlinejacc.org/cgi/content/full/44/5/1146%20

Guidelines for the Management of Patients With Peripheral Arterial Disease (Lower Extremity, Renal, Mesenteric, and Abdominal Aortic)
http://content.onlinejacc.org/cgi/content/full/47/6/1239

Guidelines for the Management of Patients With Supraventricular Arrhythmias
http://content.onlinejacc.org/cgi/content/full/42/8/1493

Guidelines for the Management of Patients With Unstable Angina/Non-ST-Segment Elevation Myocardial Infarction
http://content.onlinejacc.org/cgi/content/full/50/7/652

Guidelines for Management of Patients With Ventricular Arrhythmias and the Prevention of Sudden Cardiac Death
http://content.onlinejacc.org/cgi/content/full/48/5/1064

ACCF/AHA 2009 Expert Consensus Document on Pulmonary Hypertension: A Report of the American College of Cardiology Foundation Task Force on Clinical Expert Consensus Documents
http://content.onlinejacc.org/cgi/content/full/j.jacc.2009.01.004v1

Hypertrophic Cardiomyopathy
http://content.onlinejacc.org/cgi/content/full/42/9/1687

Tilt Table Testing for Assessing Syncope
http://www.cardiosource.org/~/media/Images/ACC/Science%20and%20Quality/Practice%20Guidelines/t/tilt.ashx

Index

Tradenames = **bold**   Active agent = *italic*

Tradenames = **bold**   Active agent = *italic*

Tradenames = **bold**   Active agent = *italic*

Tradenames = **bold**   Active agent = *italic*

Tradenames = **bold**   Active agent = *italic*

W

Z

Tradenames = bold   *Active agent = italic*

Notes

Notes

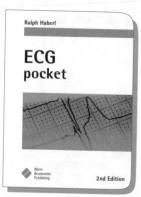
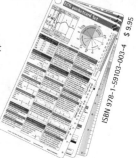

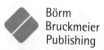

pocketcards

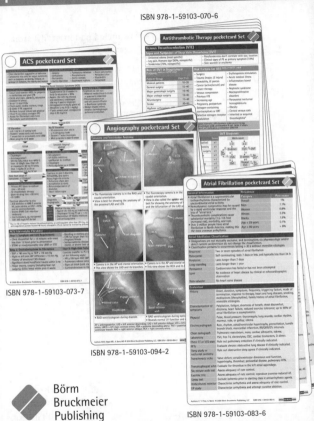

ISBN 978-1-59103-070-6

Antithrombotic Therapy pocketcard Set

ACS pocketcard Set

ISBN 978-1-59103-073-7

Angiography pocketcard Set

ISBN 978-1-59103-094-2

Atrial Fibrillation pocketcard Set

ISBN 978-1-59103-083-6

Börm
Bruckmeier
Publishing

pocketcards

ISBN 978-1-59103-071-3

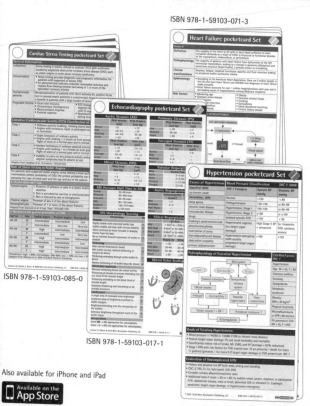

Heart Failure pocketcard Set

Cardiac Stress Testing pocketcard Set

ISBN 978-1-59103-085-0

Echocardiography pocketcard Set

ISBN 978-1-59103-017-1

Hypertension pocketcard Set

ISBN 978-1-59103-042-3

Also available for iPhone and iPad

Available on the
App Store

ECG Cases pocket

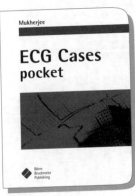

ISBN 978-1-59103-229-6
$ 16.95

- ECG Cases pocket provides 60 examples of common clinical problems encountered in the wards, emergency room, or outpatient sitting

- Each ECG is preceded by a brief clinical history and pertinent physical examination findings, so that the the tracings may be interpreted in the appropriate clinical context

- Detailed answers concentrate on the clinical interpretation of the clinical interpretation of the results and give advice on what to do

- The convinient size of this book will enable medical students, interns, residents, and other trainees to carry it in their pockets, for use as a quick reference

Börm
Bruckmeier
Publishing

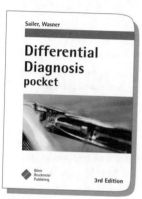

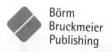

Vital Tool for Anyone Communicating with Spanish-Speaking Patients

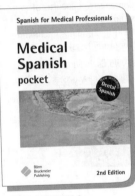

Spanish for Medical Professionals

Medical Spanish pocket

NEW INCLUDING Dental Spanish

Börm Bruckmeier Publishing

2nd Edition

ISBN 978-1-59103-232-8
$ 16.95

- 2nd edition, completely updated
- Now including: Dental Spanish
- Clearly organized by history and physical examination with specific in-depth question and phrases appropriate to each medical speciality
- Bilingual dictionary containing Spanish medical terminology specific to Mexico, Puerto Rico, Cuba, and other countries
- Provides hundreds of essential ready to use words and phrases

Börm
Bruckmeier
Publishing